NURSING RESEARCH: DESIGN AND PRACTICE

Nursing Research
Design and Practice

edited by

Margaret P. Treacy
and Abbey Hyde

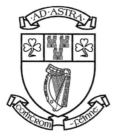

University College Dublin Press
Preas Choláiste Ollscoile Bhaile Átha Cliath

First published 1999 by University College Dublin Press
Newman House, St Stephen's Green, Dublin 2, Ireland
www.ucdpress.ie

ISBN 1 900621 29 0

Cataloguing in Publication data available from the British Library

Index by John Loftus
Typset in 11/12½ Bembo and Gill Sans by
Elaine Shiels, Bantry, Co. Cork, Ireland
Printed in Ireland by Colour Books, Dublin

Contents

Contents

Part I

Research Design

1
Contextualising Irish Nursing Research

Margaret P. Treacy and Abbey Hyde

Nursing Research: Design and Practice is the first book that deals specifically with nursing research[1] carried out in the Republic of Ireland and which presents that research in the context of methodological approaches in research. The book introduces the reader to research designs and processes and provides examples of the application of research strategies to research questions; this will facilitate readers' understanding of the research process by linking theoretical and methodological issues in research with the actual practice of research. Furthermore, in publishing studies undertaken in the Irish context within a single volume, the book presents a flavour of the current state of nursing research in Ireland. In this sense, it is not simply a text for students but part of a historical record of the development of Irish nursing research. Part I consists of seven chapters, providing an introduction to the strategies and processes of doing research; it includes chapters on qualitative and quantitative approaches, planning research, critiquing research and utilising research. Part II provides some samples of empirical work which illustrate the practical application of research strategies presented in Part I.

This introductory chapter provides a context for Parts I and II in exploring issues that are relevant to nurses and nursing students in Ireland who are studying research. It begins by considering the purpose and meaning of nursing research and follows this with an account of knowledge and skills required by practising nurses in relation to research. A brief overview of research approaches and their relationship to theory is then furnished which serves to integrate various issues in Part I of the book, while drawing on examples from Part II. Finally, the context for this book is explored in a sketch of nursing research developments in Ireland to date.

THE PURPOSE AND MEANING OF NURSING RESEARCH

Nursing research is important for the continued development of nursing practice and for some years now nurses in Ireland and elsewhere have been exhorted to develop an understanding of research and research skills (Working Party Report, 1980). More recent publications highlight research career pathways for nurses and acknowledge the importance of nursing research (An Bord Altranais, 1997; Carroll Report, 1998). The more recent emphasis on evidence-based practice in nursing further demonstrates the need for nursing practice research (Kitson, 1997). The acknowledgement of the need for establishing a knowledge base for practice is not new. In 1859, Florence Nightingale wrote:

> In dwelling upon the vital importance of sound observation it must never be lost sight of what observation is for. It is not for the sake of miscellaneous information or curious facts, but for the sake of saving life and increasing health and comfort. (Nightingale, 1859: 70)

Yet, for many years the nursing profession lost sight of the goal of research based practice. Today, the goal of nursing research remains focused on the improvement of patient care.

A debate has taken place in the past about the scope of nursing research. One perception of nursing research is that it should be confined to studies that directly relate to nursing practice (American Nurses Association, 1981: 2). In this paper it is suggested that broad definitions are more appropriate to the open spirit of enquiry necessary for the advancement of nursing research. It is further suggested that nursing research is concerned with the study of all aspects of nursing and nurses in so far as these bear a relationship to and have an impact on nursing or midwifery care delivery. Within this definition, factors such as the scope of practice, structures for care delivery, preparation for practice and all aspects of nursing care delivery regardless of setting are within the scope of the nurse researcher. In some instances, boundaries between nursing and other research may be blurred as overlaps may exist with research in other related areas. Burns and Grove (1997: 4) acknowledge the wide scope of nursing research in the following quotation:

> Nursing research is defined as a scientific process that validates and refines existing knowledge and generates new knowledge that directly and indirectly influences nursing practice.

In this volume, the papers by McCarthy and Farrelly are examples of research on clinical practice and have very direct implications for patient care. Research findings that have an indirect impact on care are reflected in the chapters by Begley, Clarke et al., O'Meara Kearney, and Treacy and Collins. Begley's study of student midwives' perceptions of their training illuminates the way in which students' experiences impacted on their role in providing midwifery care. Similarly O'Meara Kearney's exploration of nurses' perceptions of their role identifies problems in the nursing environment that nurses in the sample believed affected the quality of the care they were able to provide. Clarke et al.'s work in evaluating the Diploma in Nursing programme and Treacy's and Collins's work on nurses' understanding and practices in relation to health promotion have obvious yet indirect implications for nursing practice. These papers illustrate the importance of nursing research activities retaining a broad remit so that the delivery of nursing care and the study of factors indirectly affecting patient care are potential areas of study for the nurse researcher.

It is suggested here that broad definitions of nursing research are appropriate to the continued development of nursing research into the new millennium in Ireland, while giving primacy to the need for nurses to undertake research on topics directly affecting nursing practice. Nursing research today is considered increasingly important, with continual changes in knowledge and an increasing emphasis on evidence-based practice and quality improvement in hospitals (Titler et al., 1994). In a climate of change, it is important that the goal of nursing research remains focused on the improvement of patient care.

KNOWLEDGE AND SKILLS FOR RESEARCH

Burns and Grove (1997) suggest that the knowledge and skills needed to carry out research are the same in nursing as in other disciplines and what makes nursing research different from research in other disciplines, apart from its scope, is its incorporation of nursing values, theories and established knowledge, as appropriate, into research activities. In other words, it takes place within a context of nursing orientations and knowledge. The knowledge of research that clinical nurses and nurse managers require is referred to as research awareness or research mindedness. This differs from actually carrying out research projects; rather, clinical nurses and nurse managers are required to be critical consumers of research conducted, in most cases, by nurse researchers and others.

Hunt (1997), in the foreword to Smith's (1997) book, writes that nurses must become research minded now more than ever with the advent of 'evidence based practice'. She points out that research mindedness is a necessary part of everyday nursing care. It is important to explore what this means. Goodman (1989: 95) states: 'The research-aware nurse is one who can find and comprehend research literature and apply its findings to her area of practice.' An understanding of the term 'research awareness' is important because it can seem to refer simply to the nurses' recognition of the need for research. When the concept is examined it becomes clear that research-aware nurses need knowledge and understanding of research approaches, an ability to read research reports as well as the ability to utilise knowledge related to their area of practice. The importance of the capacity to read research is exemplified in chapter 8 where Kathy Redmond and Laserina O'Connor take the reader through a literature review which looks at the factors that influence nurses' assessment of pain. In chapter 5, Therese Connell Meehan brings the reader through the essential task that many nurses find difficult, that of critiquing research. In chapter 6, Gerard M. Fealy highlights the issues and routes to research utilisation for nurses. As nursing research has developed in other countries it has become increasingly obvious that the implementation of findings in nursing practice is a complex matter. All nurses need to be able to read and assess a research report and make some evaluation of it in relation to their practice. They also must understand issues that may affect their ability to implement it in practice.

RESEARCH, METHOD, METHODOLOGY AND THEORY

In the course of this book, it will become clear that a variety of strategies and techniques are used to develop nursing knowledge. The sheer breadth of research designs and the associated jargon that accompanies them often baffle students new to the language of research. This section presents an overview of central issues in research which are discussed further in later chapters. This provides only a starting point for novices to research, as much of the information here has been condensed and simplified.

A crude distinction between different research approaches is the divide between quantitative research and qualitative research. *Quantitative research*, as Roger Watson in chapter 4 indicates, is concerned with measurement and assigning numerical values to concepts that may be analysed using statistics. On the other hand, as Sam Porter explores in chapter 3, *qualitative research* tends to attempt to understand people's interpretations and motivations, with a focus on *words* people use as categories for analysis.

The divergence of these approaches arises from the differing way in which they relate to the natural sciences. Quantitative approaches are associated with *positivism*, that is, the adoption of the natural sciences, such as physics and chemistry, as a methodological model for developing knowledge in the social sciences – disciplines concerned with human thoughts, actions and interactions. Central to positivism is the notion that social phenomena are subject to pattern formation and deterministic laws in a similar way to those occurring in the natural sciences (Poloma,

1979). As Roger Watson's chapter indicates, in quantitative research designs, quantitatively measured variables are manipulated to identify interrelationships between phenomena.

Qualitative approaches are located within the *interpretative* school, and these question the notion of using traditional methods from the natural sciences to explain and predict human behaviour. The strategies of observation and measurement used by positivists are believed to neglect and distort the complexity of the subjective rationalities and strategies which form the basis of human social processes (Cohen, 1987). The interpretative paradigm is instead concerned with understanding human behaviour by making it intelligible and uncovering the meaning or significance of such behaviour (Rosenberg, 1988). The everyday common-sense notions of social phenomena which people hold are considered important subject matter. Interpretative methodologists assert that human behaviour cannot be reduced to the laws of natural science (Poloma, 1979).

The divide between qualitative and quantitative approaches is by no means precise, as there is a great deal of diversity within each school of thought (Atkinson, 1995), as well as overlaps between the two (Porter, 1996). Dealing with them separately simply provides a starting point for novices to research, and also assists in elucidating the relationship between research and theory. Before elaborating on this relationship, a brief account of the meanings of the terms 'method', 'methodology' and 'theory' is furnished. As with most complex and abstract notions, various meanings have been applied to these concepts in the literature.

According to Harding (1987), a research method is a mechanism for gathering data or evidence. Harding identifies three methods, namely listening to (or interrogating) subjects (for example by interview or questionnaire), observing them, or searching through historical records. In other literature, the term 'method' has been used more generally to refer to actual strategies for undertaking a research project, such as the 'grounded theory method' (Benton, 1996: 123), and indeed at a more abstract level to refer to broad research approaches such as qualitative and quantitative strategies (Field and Morse, 1985: 1). Frustrating though it may be for novices to research, there is no one meaning that is the 'right' one; however an understanding of 'method' is facilitated by associating it with the techniques and processes of gathering and analysing data.

Data-gathering instruments such as the interview can be used in many different ways; for example they can be highly structured or unstructured, with a range of variations in between. The content, structure and process of the technique (method) are determined by the *methodology* (Sarantakos, 1993: 33). As Porter (1996: 116) notes, '[m]ethodology concerns questions about the manner in which knowledge about what exists can be gained'. In a broad sense, methodologies provide research principles that influence and guide the process of research (for a useful analysis of methodologies, see Sarantakos 1993: 32). There are several methodologies, and it is useful to remember that none is written on tablets of stone. Even well-established methodologies are constantly being questioned and revised by scholars in a quest to attain the most valid knowledge about events. Individual researchers frequently adapt established methodologies in innovative ways according to the dictates of their particular projects. A case in point is Aine O'Meara Kearney's study in chapter 11 of general nurses' perceptions of their role as nurses, using a methodology in which focus group interviewing was used in conjunction with a grounded theory approach. The focus group is a relative newcomer as a data-gathering technique, and O'Meara Kearney's chapter offers readers a good description of how it merged with Glaser's and Strauss's (1967) grounded theory in the research process.

Meanings associated with the word 'theory' in research are also diverse and contentious. Sarantakos (1993: 9) suggests that an agreed definition of 'theory' among many methodologists is to view it as 'a set of systematically tested and logically interrelated propositions that have been developed through research and that explain social phenomena'. He considers that this definition is more closely aligned with quantitative work. Field and Morse (1985: 3), who are strongly associated with qualitative scholarship, define theory as 'the researcher's perception of reality in which constructs and concepts are identified and relationships are proposed or predictions made. It is a systematic explanation of an event'. Clearly, according to such definitions, theory is associated with 'propositions' and the 'perceptions of reality' of the theorist, or, loosely speaking, his or her interpretation and explanation of events, supported by evidence. It has been argued that constructing theory is not the objective of all research; some projects aim instead to describe or classify rather than theorise (Sarantakos, 1993: 9). Also, methodologies that draw on phenomenology do not seek to develop abstract theories but rather to uncover the meaning in lived experiences.

Theory has also been conceptualised into different types such as deductive or inductive, according to the type of reasoning upon which it draws. *Deductive theories* are framed from existing knowledge and potential relationships are deduced from this knowledge base. The starting point in deductive theorising is a set of concepts or conceptual framework. The researcher formulates a hypothesis based on existing knowledge that he or she then tests out. In the case of *inductive reasoning*, the theoretical insights are inductively derived from the data generated; it is the data that determine what theoretical insights are generated. While quantitative work is closely associated with deductive theorising, and qualitative work with inductive theorising, many research projects draw on both types of reasoning at different points of the research process (see, for example, Aine O'Meara Kearney's account in chapter 11 of the process of generating theoretical insights from data, and later testing these with data, using grounded theory).

The relationship between method and theory becomes clearer when methodology is considered. Certain philosophical assumptions and theoretical perspectives about what counts as knowledge mediate methodologies and the way in which knowledge can be developed. These philosophical premises and theoretical foundations in turn may affect the findings of the study, because the use of an alternative research strategy with a contrasting set of assumptions and so forth may have yielded different data. Since data are closely linked with the interpretation offered and/or theoretical insights generated, theories and beliefs cross-cutting the process of research in turn may impact upon theories and propositions emanating from the research.

In broad terms, diverse assumptions underpinning qualitative and quantitative methodologies have been identified (Guba and Lincoln, 1994). Methodologies associated with the interpretative paradigm assert that theory and facts are interdependent, in so far as it is within a particular theoretical framework that facts actually become facts. This undermines the objectivity of facts, and contrasts with positivist approaches, which assume that theory and fact are separate in the testing of hypotheses (Guba and Lincoln, 1994). Furthermore, in the interpretative school it is deemed that different theoretical frameworks may well be supported by the same 'facts'. It recognises that, just as theories and facts are not separate, neither are values and facts – values are seen to mediate theoretical positions. This challenges the positivist position that knowledge should be value-free. Moreover, within the interpretative approach, it is acknowledged that the interactive nature of the researcher/participant relationship has the potential to shape the study outcome; this challenges the notion of objectivity claimed by positivists (Guba and Lincoln, 1994).

These differences in assumptions between the two schools lend themselves to different conduct in the research process. For example, in using the interview method, positivist researchers tend to favour a highly structured approach, because they believe that this increases objectivity and reduces the risk of bias by the interviewer. Interpretative researchers tend to allow a lot more leeway to interviewees in order to gain rich data, and accept that subjectivity is a feature of interaction in the interview setting. The volume and quality of the data obtained are most likely to be affected by each of these strategies. In the case of the former, greater consistency in data is likely in so far as all participants will have been asked exactly the same questions, but the degree of depth in responses is compromised. In the case of the latter, richer data of uneven quality and quantity is more likely, as well as constraints in terms of generalisability of findings because of the tendency to use smaller sample sizes. The style of analysis in both cases will differ, and all of this ultimately impacts on the findings.

Mary Farrelly's qualitative study in chapter 9 of the experiences of in-patients of a psychiatric hospital clearly demonstrates how Streubert's (1991) phenomenological approach led to the development of rich data on the subject matter under investigation. Farrelly notes that previous research on the topic used quantitative designs, which constrained individuals' responses to those amenable to quantitative measurement, thus limiting the depth that could be achieved. However, Farrelly acknowledges that while depth was achieved in relation to her findings, the small sample size limited the study's scope and generalisability.

It is not so much that contradictory findings are a likely outcome – although this is, of course, a possibility – of using very different research approaches, but rather that the emphasis varies. The lack of depth in responses may limit theoretical insights of the quantitative researcher, while the lack of empirical scope may hinder interpretations of the qualitative researcher. Different methodologies guiding the same research question can of course produce consistent findings and the weaknesses of one strategy may be compensated by the strengths of the other. The qualitative component may yield rich data but is restricted in terms of generalisability, while the quantitative component may lack depth and richness, yet allow generalisations to be made. As Parahoo and McKenna note in chapter 2, the choice of approach depends largely on the research question and the purpose of the study.

The notion of mixing research strategies within the same study is referred to as triangulation. This strategy was used by Cecily Begley (see chapter 14) in her research into midwifery training. In Begley's study, two questionnaires comprised the quantitative component: one was administered at the outset of the student midwives' training, and one at the end, with both individual and focus group interviews generating qualitative data. The second questionnaire was constructed on the basis of qualitative data gleaned, and findings from the qualitative aspect supported those of the quantitative component.

NURSING RESEARCH IN IRELAND

Lest it be misunderstood, nursing research in Ireland has not begun with the publication of the chapters in this volume; rather the work included represents part of the culmination of the work of the previous generation of nurses who advocated research awareness among nurses. The Irish Nursing Research Interest Group, the Faculty of Nursing, Royal College of

Surgeons in Ireland (RCSI), An Bord Altranais and the Department of Nursing Studies (now School of Nursing and Midwifery) at University College Dublin (UCD) all played an important role in generating awareness, delivering courses in research and supporting nurses in their research endeavours.

The provision of education in research approaches was left largely to third-level institutions, most particularly the Faculty of Nursing, RCSI, which from the late 1970s ran short diploma courses in research methods for nurses. These courses were also extended to some of the regions through a system of local centres. Outside the higher education sector An Bord Altranais also provided short research appreciation courses. Courses were also provided as part of in-service education programmes.

In University College Dublin, 'research methods' was introduced as a subject on the nurse tutors' diploma programme and this was extended to include a dissertation under supervision when it became a degree programme in 1984. Apart from these courses, which focused specifically on nursing, a small number of nurses have obtained degrees at Master's level in disciplines such as education, psychology and sociology. This gave those nurses varying levels of expertise in research approaches and usually allowed them to undertake small pieces of research under supervision. In January 1992, the UCD Bachelor of Nursing Studies programme was expanded to meet the needs of clinical nurses and was offered on a part-time basis. The Faculty of Nursing, RCSI, commenced a similar part-time programme in October 1994. Since then many other institutions have followed suit and there is a greater availability of degree programmes for registered nurses. The current ongoing development of Diploma/Registration programmes present more opportunities for the creation and development of research awareness in student nurses.

Although there is no cause for complacency, progress has been made in research education for nurses. This can be measured by considering the development of postgraduate studies. By 1980, one nurse in this country had obtained a PhD (Scanlon, 1966). Another PhD thesis was completed in 1987 (Treacy, 1987), and, since then, four others have been completed (McCarthy, 1993; Cowman, 1994; Hyde, 1996; Begley, 1997). Initially, nurses who pursued higher education tended to have a background in education. However, the current Master of Science (Nursing/Midwifery) in UCD offers three optional strands in clinical, management and educational studies. In 1999 in Ireland, studies are available at Master's and PhD levels in nursing. As opportunities for studies at postgraduate level in nursing and midwifery continue to expand, more research will emerge. For nursing research to develop in Ireland work needs to be undertaken under supervision at Master's and PhD levels and independently at post-doctoral level.

To date many nurses in Ireland have undertaken courses in research and are to some degree research aware. However this has been achieved with a small amount of organisational support and a lot of personal motivation, financing, and commitment on the part of nurses themselves. Educational programmes and research activity need to continue to be developed and funding is required.

Funding for Research

The nursing service constitutes a large part of the health service in Ireland. Because of its potential one would assume that appropriate funding for the development of that service would be made available. Yet, apart from An Bord Altranais's important provision of library services and its most recent establishment of scholarships for doctoral studies, funding provided from central and other sources has tended to be for one-off research projects. Examples of such projects include Hanrahan's (1968) work funded by the Irish Matrons' Association, McGowan's (1979) study of nurses' attitudes funded by the Department of Health, research on nurse staffing by Treacy (1988) and Treacy (1990) funded by the Irish Matrons' Association and the Department of Health respectively, and Wynne et al.'s (1993) work on stress and nursing which was funded by the Irish Nurses' Organisation.[2] The Department of Health has funded a small number of studies but this research has been one-off and not part of an overall nursing research programme. It has also provided some funding for other ad hoc isolated projects (Research and Development posts) and Practice Development Coordinators which can contribute to the development of research and/or research-based practice. In addition to the foregoing, nurses have access to small bursaries which can assist towards studies or small research projects. In general the development and promotion of nursing research have been left almost entirely in the hands of the nursing profession at the level of education programme provision.

Funding for nursing research is also available from the Health Research Board and the National Rehabilitation Board.[3] These organisations provide financial support for postgraduate studies and larger-scale projects. Until recently, nurses were free to apply for funding but had to compete with other professionals for resources. However, a significant new development announced in Spring of 1999 is the availability of research fellowships by the Health Research Board specifically for clinical nursing and midwifery research. While this funding appears to be restrictive in terms of the substantive areas for study (clinical realms), it is nonetheless a major step forward in the provision of financial support for nursing research.

In addition to securing financial support for research, nurses also need opportunities to work in nursing research centres to further develop their expertise and research agendas. The continued establishment of nursing studies within the higher education sector will assist the process. Given its embryonic state and a need to undertake research involving both qualitative and qualitative designs, it is essential that this funding is exclusively made available for nursing research as defined in its widest sense.

In Ireland, the movement that exists for nursing research is essentially one that is driven by the nursing profession. While this is important it also has disadvantages; an absence of central funding has meant that no coherent planned approach has been taken to the development of nursing research. Researchers have tended to pursue personal interests or undertaken fragmented pieces of research on isolated topics depending on the availability of funding. The papers presented in Part II of this book are an outcome of these circumstances. They cover a range of interests and study designs. In terms of research strategies they are representative of both qualitative and quantitative research, albeit the emphasis on qualitative research approaches is apparent and is a reflection of trends in nursing and health research. This developing strength in the field of qualitative research strategies should be built upon. In addition, it is important to continue the application of quantitative research methodologies to nursing problems.

Nursing research in Ireland is at a different stage in its development from nursing research in the United Kingdom. Irish nursing shares similar concerns in relation to methodologies best suited to the study of nursing, issues in relation to research education for nurses, gaps in research on nursing practice and the utilisation of research findings. However, the base from which nurses in Ireland are now attempting to develop research-based practice is different in terms of the absence of funding and organisational support. In order to expand nursing research further and build on the type of work represented in this volume, it is essential that these constraints be addressed.

NOTES

1 The term nursing research is used throughout this chapter. It is used as an inclusive term and refers also to midwifery research.
2 The work indicated here is not a comprehensive list of work funded but is an indication of the piecemeal ad hoc nature of funding for research on nursing issues.
3 Funding is also available through the European Union

REFERENCES

American Nurses Association (1981) *Research Priorities for the 1980s: Generating a Scientific Basis for Nursing Practice*. Commission on Nursing Research. Kansas MO: American Nurses Association.

Atkinson, P. (1995) Pearls, pith, and provocation: some perils of paradigms, *Qualitative Health Research*, 5 (1): 117–24.

Begley, C.M. (1997) 'Midwives in the making: a longitudinal study of the experiences of student midwives during their two year training in Ireland', Unpublished PhD thesis, University of Dublin, Trinity College.

Benton, D.C. (1996) Grounded theory, in: D. Cormac (ed.), *The Research Process in Nursing* (3rd edn). London: Blackwell: 123–34

An Bord Altranais (1997) *Continuing Professional Education for Nurses in Ireland: A Framework*. Dublin: An Bord Altranais (The Nursing Board).

Burns, N. and Grove, S. K. (1997) *The Practice of Nursing Research: Conduct, Critique, and Utilization* (3rd edn). Philadelphia: W.B. Saunders.

Carroll Report (1998) *Report of the Commission on Nursing: A Blueprint for the Future*. Dublin: Stationery Office.

Cohen, I.J. (1987) Structuration theory and social praxis, in: A. Giddens and J. H. Turner (eds), *Social Theory Today*. Cambridge: Polity: 273–301.

Cowman, S. (1994) 'Understanding Student Nurse Learning', Unpublished PhD thesis, Dublin City University.

Field P. A. and Morse, J. M. (1985) *Nursing Research: The Application of Qualitative Approaches*. London: Chapman & Hall.

Glaser, B.G. and Strauss, A.L. (1967) *The Discovery of Grounded Theory: Strategies for Qualitative Research*. Chicago: Aldine.

Goodman, C. (1989) Nursing research: growth and development, in: M. Jolley and P. Allen (eds), *Current Issues in Nursing*. London: Chapman Hall: 95–114.

Guba, E. and Lincoln, Y. (1994) Competing paradigms in qualitative research, in: N. Denzin and Y. Lincoln (eds), *Handbook of Qualitative Research*. London: Sage: 105–17.

Hanrahan, E. (1968) *Report on the Training of Student Nurses*. Dublin: Irish Matrons Association.

Harding, S. (1987) Is there a feminist methodology?, in: S. Harding (ed.), *Feminism and Methodology: Social Science Issues*. Milton Keyes: Open University Press: 1–14.

Hunt, J.M. (1997) Foreword, in: P. Smith, *Research Mindedness for Practice*. New York: Churchill Livingstone.

Hyde, A. (1996) 'Unmarried Women's Experiences of Pregnancy and the Early Weeks of Motherhood in an Irish Context: A Qualitative Analysis', Unpublished PhD thesis, University of Dublin, Trinity College.

Kitson, A. (1997) Using evidence to demonstrate the value of nursing, *Nursing Standard*, 11 (28): 34–9.

McCarthy, G. (1993) 'Cognitive Appraisal, Coping Responses, Social Support and Psycho-social Adjustment in Irish Women with Breast Cancer Receiving Psychotoxic Chemotherapy', Unpublished PhD thesis, Case Western Reserve University.

McGowan, J. (1979) *Attitude Survey of Irish Nurses*. Dublin: Institute of Public Administration.

Nightingale, Florence (1859) *Notes on Nursing: what it is, and what it is not*. Facsimile reprint (undated). London: Harrison/Philadelphia: J.B. Lippincott.

Poloma, M. (1979) *Contemporary Sociological Theory*. London: Collier Macmillan.

Porter, S. (1996) Qualitative research, in: D. Cormac (ed.), *The Research Process in Nursing* (3rd edn). London: Blackwell: 113–22.

Rosenberg, A. (1988) *Philosophy and Social Science*. Oxford: Clarendon.

Sarantakos, S. (1993) *Social Research*. London: Macmillan.

Scanlon, P. (1966) 'Nursing Education in Ireland, Background, Present Status and Future', Unpublished PhD thesis, Washington DC: Catholic University of America.

Smith, P. (1997) *Research Mindedness for Practice*. New York: Churchill Livingstone.

Streubert, H.J. (1991) Phenomenologic research as a theoretic initiative in community health nursing, *Public Health Nursing*, 8 (2): 119–23.

Titler, M. G., Kleiber, C., Steelman,V., Goode, C., Rakel, B., Barry-Walker, J., Small, S., and Buckwalter, K. (1994) Infusing research into practice to promote quality care, *Nursing Research*, 43 (5): 307–13.

Treacy, M. (1987) '"In the Pipeline": A Qualitative Study of General Nurse Training with Special Reference to Nurses' Role in Health Education', PhD thesis, University of London.

Treacy, M. (1988) *Setting Establishments in Nursing – A Pilot Study*. Dublin: Irish Matrons' Association.

Treacy, M. (1990) *A Study of Establishment Setting in Selected Medical and Surgical Wards in St James' Hospital, Dublin*. Dublin: St James' Hospital/Department of Health.

Working Party on General Nursing (1980), *Working Party on General Nursing Report*. Dublin: Department of Health.

Wynne, R., Clarkin, N., and McNieve, A. (1993) *The Experience of Stress Amongst Irish Nurses: A Survey of Irish Nurses' Organisation Members, Main Report*. Work Research Centre, Dublin: Irish Nurses' Organisation.

2
Planning a Research Study

Kader Parahoo and Hugh McKenna

INTRODUCTION

Planning a research project primarily requires a knowledge of the principles, process and issues underpinning research. You must be able to demonstrate careful thinking about all the steps and decisions you intend to take in carrying out your proposed study. In this chapter, you will learn about the importance of prior preparation as well as the actual plan for your project. Methodological, practical, ethical and other aspects will be highlighted.

You must be able to explain clearly, in advance, what is to be researched, the methods of data collection and analysis and the resources required for such an undertaking. Clarity, attention to detail and logical thinking are some of the key criteria by which a plan is evaluated. You must also demonstrate awareness and insight into what your particular project will involve.

Research and Nursing Practice

Every profession needs a body of knowledge on which to base its practice (McKenna, 1997). This comes mainly from experience and research. There is an increasing realisation that many nursing practices are not underpinned by sound evidence. Research has the potential to provide a solid knowledge base for nursing practice by seeking answers to some of the questions posed by practitioners and others. These questions emanate from experience, reading the literature and/or talking to patients and other professionals.

The generation of a knowledge base comes about through the study of phenomena using rigorous and systematic approaches to the collection of data (Parahoo, 1997: 10). Nursing is a young discipline and therefore many of the phenomena with which nurses deal have yet to be explored, developed and verified. The recent drive towards evidence based practice in the health sector has once again highlighted the importance of research to practice (Parahoo, 1997: 10).

The emphasis here is on using available research findings after systematically reviewing them. Nonetheless, there is also a need for primary research as many clinical practices in nursing remain un-researched or under-researched.

THE IMPORTANCE OF PLANNING

A research plan is a tool for articulating on paper and in a structured way the thoughts and decisions of the researcher. It is also a way of checking that everything has been well thought out in advance and that nothing has been left to chance. A good plan is clear, comprehensive, logical and realistic. The culmination of a coherent plan is a quality research proposal.

A plan is useful for several reasons. First, it helps you to clarify your ideas and decisions. It also highlights the task ahead, the difficulties and issues you may encounter and gives you the opportunity to assess the feasibility of your project in relation to resources, especially time, money and expertise. Furthermore, it is helpful to others, such as ethical committee members, nurse managers, project supervisors and funding bodies who need to understand what your project involves and how you intend to carry it out.

An analogy can be drawn between planning for a research project and planning to construct a house. The builder must be able to describe and detail clearly what type of house is to be built, for example the number of rooms and other specifications. He has to assess the amount of material and the expertise required and the financial and other constraints he will have to work under. He also has to know where and when the house is to be built and the legal and practical implications. Every step, from building the foundation to painting the house must be costed. A clear and detailed building plan will inspire more confidence in house buyers than if the builder is vague and keeps most of the important information in his own head. Similarly, researchers must not only be able to write a detailed plan but must also explain and justify it.

Setting the Parameters

Research projects vary in scope and size and these depend on why they are undertaken, the funds, expertise and time available. For many of you, the reason for doing a research project will be to fulfil the requirement of a course. In this case it is likely that the project will be small and that you will be the only person doing it, albeit with some help from your supervisor. Your time, resources and research skills will be limited.

When you decide on a project you must bear these factors in mind throughout the planning process. This applies also to larger projects involving more funds or more than one researcher. It is better to over-estimate the size of the undertaking and the time and other resources required than to find that you have been over optimistic.

QUANTITATIVE RESEARCH

Planning the Project

Knowing what the parameters are only sets the context in which the project is to be carried out. You still need to know where to begin. The quantitative research process can provide a guide or structure to your plan. Although qualitative research is more flexible and less predictable, it still requires planning (this will be dealt with later on in this chapter).

The research process in quantitative research consists mainly of the following steps:

- Identifying a topic
- Formulating a research question
- Deciding the research methodology (including selecting the research approach, methods of data collection, samples and sampling, techniques of data analysis)
- Piloting instruments to be used in the study
- Collecting data
- Analysing and interpreting data
- Writing up the report.

The number of steps varies according to which textbook you read, but essentially the research process consists of three stages: formulating a research question, collection of data and analysis of data. In this chapter we will use the steps of the research process to guide you through the plan.

Identifying a topic
Students doing a research project will sometimes say that they want to do a qualitative study or they want to use questionnaires. By doing so they are clearly putting the 'cart before the horse'. Approaches and methods must suit the research question or aim, not the other way around. In essence, research methods are like the tools of your trade. Depending on what you wish to find out will determine the tool to be used. For some research questions you will go to your metaphorical tool bag and select a qualitative approach, for other questions a quantitative approach will be the tool of choice.

Research starts with a hunch or a niggling clinical question. For example, a nurse may want to know whether patients in a care of the elderly ward are satisfied with the care they receive. Another nurse may be curious about the effectiveness of diet in reducing constipation. On the other hand, students may have a topic in mind but may not know exactly what aspect of the topic to investigate. If the topic is asthma care, there are a number of aspects that can be researched such as: How do patients experience the care they receive for asthma? Do nurses have the skills and knowledge to care for asthma patients? What is the knowledge of patients of the side effects and other implications of the drugs they take for asthma? For small projects it is not possible to answer all of these questions. You have to select one that can be researched within the time and resources available to you.

Topics can be identified through reading the literature or talking to others. However, invariably they originate from clinical experience. According to McKenna (1997) research should emanate from practice and return to inform practice. Once you have an idea, it is advisable to carry out a preliminary search of the literature to find out how much is known on the topic. You will therefore be able to identify gaps in knowledge, which your research may seek to fill.

Formulating a research question
Once a topic has been identified, the next step is to formulate a clear, concise and researchable research question. Not all questions are researchable. For example, no amount of research can answer the question: should elderly care receive more funds? or should euthanasia be legalised? The first is a political question and the second, a moral question. We can, however, find out if more money is spent on acute than on elderly services or whether nurses think more money should be spent on elderly care. Similarly, we may find out if the public approves of the legalisation of euthanasia or if there is a difference between nurses' and doctors' perceptions of euthanasia. Therefore, you must not only be clear in setting your question but it must also be possible to research it.

Asking a question is only one format in which to state what is being researched. This can also be stated in the form of aims and objectives or as hypotheses. An example of an aim of a study could be 'to describe the nursing care given to patients with leg ulcers'. Because 'nursing care is a broad concept' comprising many aspects, it is important to specify which particular aspects of care the researcher wants to focus upon. Therefore, objectives can be formulated to explain further the aim of the study. Objectives are the steps the researcher must take to achieve the aim. For the above study, the objectives could be:

(*a*) To find out how nurses assess the care that patients with leg ulcers require.
(*b*) To identify the treatments nurses use for ulcers.

(*c*) To observe if, and how, nurses attend to the psychological needs of patients who have leg ulcers.

It is not possible with small projects to study all aspects of nursing care of patients who have leg ulcers. Therefore, depending on the size of the project, the researcher must necessarily be selective as to what aspects will be studied. The choice may depend on the interest of the researcher, but a rationale must be provided for the selection.

Setting hypotheses is more suited to research that investigates cause and effect. For example, a researcher may want to find out if cognitive behaviour therapy is effective in the treatment of depression. The hypothesis can be stated as follows: there will be a reduction in depression among elderly women following a course of cognitive behaviour therapy. To be complete, a hypothesis must identify the independent variable (causing the change, in this case, a course of cognitive behaviour therapy), the dependent variable (being changed, in this case depression) and the population taking part in the study (elderly women).

In formulating the purpose of a study it is important to define operationally the terms used in the questions, aims or hypothesis. In the previous example, the researcher must have a definition of depression as he or she intends to use it in this particular study. He or she may decide to use a medical diagnosis or may want to use scores on the Beck Depression Scale (Beck et al., 1961). The terms 'elderly women' and 'cognitive behaviour therapy' must also be defined precisely.

While the formulation of clear questions, aims, objectives or hypotheses is the foundation of a good quantitative study, there is no need to state the purpose of a study in more than one format. In other words, if questions are set, then hypotheses are not required. However, without a clear purpose, the study should go no further.

Deciding the research methodology
Once the research question has been formulated, you should decide how to collect and analyse data in a systematic and rigorous manner. This means taking decisions regarding which methods can best answer the research questions, achieve the aims or test the hypotheses. At this stage you must decide whether a quantitative, qualitative or a combination of these approaches would be suitable. This, in turn, depends on the type of design selected. If the data required are of a descriptive, quantitative type, then a survey may be most suitable. When the purpose is to test the effectiveness of, or compare interventions, then an experimental design is recommended. On the other hand, when in–depth exploration of a topic is the purpose of a study, then a qualitative approach such as a case study design may be best indicated.

The next step is to choose methods to collect the necessary data. The main methods in quantitative research are questionnaires, interviews and observations. The selection of one or more of these methods depends on how appropriate they are in answering the research question and through reading about how the same or similar topics have been researched. If, for example, you decide to research the attitudes of nurses towards AIDS patients, you should find out if similar studies have been carried out and decide whether their methods can be used in your study. If attitude scales for such studies have been developed already, you may find them useful, but you must seek permission prior to using them. Initial telephone enquiries are advised as this process can take weeks and often involves payment of a fee.

If there are no studies on 'nurses' attitudes to AIDS patients', you can learn from the methodology of other attitude studies such as 'nurses' attitudes to older patients'. A review of the literature is useful in giving you tips on how to carry out your own study and on some of the pitfalls you wish to avoid. You may also want to make personal contact with researchers who have published on or researched the topic already.

If you decide to construct your own data collection tools (questionnaires, interview or observation schedules), you must bear in mind that this process is also time consuming and potentially problematic. A questionnaire may require 8–12 drafts before it can be used (Crossby et al., 1989). Reliability and validity are important for any measurement tool. Validity means the instrument measures what it sets out to measure, and reliability means that it does so consistently. For instance, if you stepped onto a weighing machine and it told you what was in your bank account – it would not be valid. If you stepped on it and the first time it indicated nine stones and two minutes later it indicated fifteen stones – then it may be valid but it was not reliable.

To ensure that a questionnaire is valid and reliable, it will need to be evaluated by experienced researchers and clinicians to find out if it addresses your research question adequately (content validity). The questionnaire will also have to be tested with a small group of respondents to find out if they understand the questions and what they thought of the questionnaire generally. This 'dress rehearsal' process is called piloting. For a small project, these two strategies will be adequate to ensure validity and reliability of the instrument. For larger surveys, other more complex tests will need to be performed.

Choosing a sample

Research data are normally collected by asking people questions and/or observing phenomena. Diaries, patients/clients notes and other recording documents are also useful sources of research information – although there are ethical and legal implications in accessing and using them. If you are collecting data from people, you need to know who they are, how many to select, how to get access to them and what practical or other implications there are to obtaining the information from these sources.

In the previous example of a study on attitudes of 'Nurses towards AIDS Patients', you must define operationally the term 'nurses'. You may decide that 'nurses' in this case mean only those who are 'first level trained nurses with one year's experience of working with AIDS patients'. As you can see, this is not a dictionary definition of 'nurses' but one that suits the purpose of your study. The sample size will be decided by the availability of such nurses, the scope of the project and the statistical tests (for a quantitative study) you intend to carry out. In the latter case, you should consult a statistician who will advise you on the size of the sample, the appropriate tests and on how to code your questionnaire, interview schedule or observation schedule in order to facilitate computer data processing and analysis later on. It is wise to approach a statistician before the data have been collected; if this is left until afterwards, it may be too late for them to offer constructive advice on data analysis.

In planning your project you must pay particular attention to how you will ensure that the participants' rights are not violated or that they do not come to any harm. All research involving patients requires approval from a research ethics committee. Ethical committees would look for evidence that you have carefully considered all the ethical aspects of your proposed study. Ethical committees sometimes meet only four times per year and to avoid wasting time it is important to know when meetings take place and what the members require in order to make a judgement as to the ethical integrity of your proposed study.

Gaining ethical approval does not mean that access to potential participants is granted. Ethical committees are concerned mainly with the ethical aspects of the research and they have no control over the clinical areas where the research is to be undertaken. However, they can sometimes make valuable comments on the project. It is advisable to seek advice from 'gatekeepers' (nurse managers, doctors etc.) before making formal requests for permission to approach your sample. Such requests need time to be considered and although you are ready and keen to start collecting data, others may have their own pressing agenda. When access is finally granted, your next task is to select your sample.

Finding up-to-date lists of potential respondents/participants is another task to which you must attend. From these lists, the final sample can be selected. In turn, those approached must give their informed consent before taking part. This means that potential participants must be fully informed of the purpose and rationale of the project and what participation involves, including the benefits and possible side effects.

This information should normally be provided in writing and potential participants must be given time to consider it. It must be free of professional or other jargon and must be fully comprehensible to all people. They should also be informed of their rights to withdraw participation at any time during the project.

Collecting data

Several issues related to the collection of data need to be considered at the planning stage. For a small project, it is likely that one person will collect all the data. For larger projects, a number of researchers may be employed who will have to be briefed and, in some cases, trained for this purpose. If there is more than one data collector, measures of inter-rater reliability must be taken. This could mean finding out the degree of consistency with which they use the instruments (e.g. questionnaires, scales, interviews or observation schedules). This is to avoid different interpretation of items on the questionnaire and different interpretations of the same response or observed behaviour.

Thought should also be given to the location of the participants, the number of visits required, the mode and costs of travelling. Researchers need to be realistic concerning the number of respondents they can question or observe in one day. It may not be possible to know this at the planning stage but it is safer to keep this figure low. In any case, proper piloting of the research method will give an indication of the number of participants and the best time to contact them. More than one visit may be required. In the case of postal questionnaires, decisions will have to be taken as to the number of reminders to be sent.

Many potential respondents may be reluctant to give their opinion if they think that their response can be traced back to them. One way of assuring anonymity with questionnaires is to send out a postcard with the questionnaire. The postcard is stamped and addressed to the researcher and contains the name of the respondent plus a tick-box. When the respondents return the questionnaire they also return (separately) the postcard with a tick indicating that the questionnaire has been returned. By looking at which postcards have not been returned, the researcher can identify who has not completed the questionnaire and a reminder can be sent to them. This process ensures that all the questionnaires returned are totally anonymous and responses are confidential.

Particular times in the year are contra-indicated for data collection. During the Christmas period and in the summer time, participants are either busy or not available. Consideration should also be given as to how the data will be recorded and stored. If tape recorders are to be used, the equipment and the number of tapes required will have to be costed. It also is advisable to find out the potential costs of employing a secretary to transcribe taped interviews.

Analysing data and writing up the report

Although this phase of a project comes at the end, it requires prior planning. It is not uncommon to find that some researchers do not know what to do with the data they have collected. In quantitative research, as explained earlier, prior thought as to the statistical tests to be carried out and the statistical package to use (e.g. SPSS) must be given before the data collection takes place. If the questionnaire is coded properly before being administered to respondents, the task of data processing (i.e. feeding them into the computer), should be straightforward, although time consuming. Data processing is not difficult, but some basic training is required. On the other hand, if the project has been properly costed and funded an experienced processor can be hired.

Once the data have been analysed and interpreted, it remains to write the report. If the study is part of a course, the word limit will be stipulated. Writing up a study, whatever its size, takes more time than one expects. And, as it often happens, the submission deadline is upon you before you realise it. Normally a number of drafts are written before the final report emerges, so give yourself plenty of time to write it up and to have it typed, proof-read and presented. Tables, figures and references need special attention. The cost of typing a report can come as a shock, so get estimates beforehand.

PLANNING A QUALITATIVE PROJECT

Most of the aspects of planning quantitative projects apply to qualitative ones as well. However, since the qualitative research process is more flexible, it is not easy to plan the steps with precision and certainty. This does not mean that you have no idea of how you intend to proceed. You must provide as much information as possible. Normally the purpose of a qualitative study is to explore phenomena from the respondents' perception and experience. For example, you may decide to find out how older people live with a chronic condition such as rheumatism. The first phase is to select an appropriate method from a range of qualitative approaches such as ethnography, phenomenology or grounded theory.

The selected approach influences the choice of data collection method/s and the sampling technique. For example, if ethnography is used, the main method is participant observation and interviews (formal and informal). You should decide how long you intend to do the 'fieldwork' (the time spent collecting information in the natural living or working environment of the participants). Normally, the samples used in qualitative research are small. While the final size may not be known until the project is completed, qualitative researchers are often asked to give an indication of the number of participants they wish to interview or observe. Qualitative researchers can increase or reduce their sample according to whether they need more information or whether they keep receiving the same information (known as saturation of data).

In planning a qualitative project, you must therefore have an idea of the initial size of your sample and make some allowance for the possibility that this may increase slightly. The number of visits to respondents should also be planned and careful budgeting should be undertaken to meet the cost of travelling and other expenses.

Data collection is more in-depth in qualitative than in quantitative studies. Interviews can last from half an hour to two hours. The method of recording can be decided in advance. If you decide to use a tape recorder, you may wish to consider whether it should be a large or a small machine and whether it should be on the table in front of the respondent or out of sight. You should make sure you have spare tapes and batteries if required and that the respondents' fears about confidentiality of taped material are assuaged. Such ethical issues are extremely important.

The cost of translating data can be more costly than in quantitative research, and the time taken to analyse and interpret the results can be longer. To ensure rigour, transcripts are often read by other researchers for the purpose of 'validating' the data. At the planning stage, you should have an idea of whom to approach for validation and give them plenty of time to expect the arrival of the scripts. The process of writing up the report is no less painful and time consuming than in quantitative research. Therefore the same advice, given earlier, applies.

Overall, although the qualitative research process is more unpredictable than the quantitative one, it also requires careful planning. Researchers are expected to give as much information as possible in their proposals for funding agencies to decide whether they will finance the project or not.

SUMMARY AND CONCLUSIONS

In this chapter the importance of planning a project has been highlighted. In particular, researchers have to be clear about what is being researched, why the research is necessary and how the study is to be carried out. Other issues such as the time, location, ethical implications, practical problems and resource allocation must also be considered. Although arduous, this exercise will make you more confident and make others (who may read your proposal) realise how serious and informed you are about your project.

It is not possible to predict with precision how a project will develop and the best planning will not avert all the problems that may arise. Poor planning, on the other hand, is a recipe for disaster. The old adage applies: those who fail to plan, plan to fail.

REFERENCES

Beck, A.T., Ward, C.H., Mendelson, M., Mock, J., and Erbaugh, J. (1961) Inventory for measuring depression, *Archives of General Psychiatry*, 4: 53–63.

Crossby, F.E., Ventura, M.R., and Feldman, M.J. (1989) Examination of a survey methodology: Dillman's design method, *Nursing Research*, 38 (1): 56–8.

McKenna, H.P. (1997) *Nursing Models and Theories*. London: Routledge.

Parahoo, K. (1997) *Nursing Research: Principles, Process and Issues*. Basingstoke: Macmillan.

3

Qualitative Research

Sam Porter

LOCATING QUALITATIVE RESEARCH

Before examining qualitative research in detail, we need to ask what it is and what makes it different from other forms of research. The short answer to these questions is that the qualitative research differs from most other forms of research in that, instead of focusing primarily upon the identification and explanation of facts, it seeks to uncover people's interpretations of those facts. Thus, qualitative research has a specific subject matter; unlike quantitative research which can examine, for example, molecules, planets, humans or plants, qualitative research is solely concerned with the study of thinking human beings. Put another way, qualitative research is an appropriate mode of enquiry when researchers wish to study the understandings and motivations that lead people to act in the way that they do. These rather sweeping statements require clarification. First of all, we need to understand what is meant by the terms 'quantitative' and 'qualitative' research and how they differ.

COMPARING QUALITATIVE AND QUANTITATIVE RESEARCH

The first difference that can be noted between quantitative and qualitative research is the focus of their analysis. While the focus of quantitative research is primarily upon *numbers*, often analysed by the use of statistics, qualitative research concentrates on *words*, either in the form of speech or writing. In this chapter, I will focus on speech and conversation, though you should be aware that it is possible to apply qualitative methods to the analysis of documents.

In addition to their focus of analysis, each approach is associated with a number of assumptions. Quantitative methods are often associated with the aim of identifying and explaining 'cause and effect' relationships. Thus, by noting that apples always fell to the ground when loosened from a tree, Newton argued that this constant conjunction of events must be the result of a cause and effect relationship. By propounding his law of gravity, he explained the relationship. In other words, gravity caused the constant effect of apples falling towards the earth when they were no longer attached to a tree.

Qualitative researchers often argue that this sort of explanation is inappropriate when the subject matter of research is the actions of thinking human beings. Apples have no choice but to fall to the ground; indeed, because apples are incapable of thought, it makes no sense to think of what happens to them in terms of choice. In contrast, human beings often do have a choice about the sort of behaviour they display; their capacity to choose being based upon their capacity to think about things, and specifically to think about the options open to them given their circumstances and desires. As a consequence, it is argued that research into human behaviour, rather than regarding it as the result of outside causal processes, should focus on the motivations that people have for doing the sorts of things that they do. In short, qualitative research is often associated with the search for reasons rather than causes. This, in turn, means that, in contrast to quantitative methods, whose aim is often to *explain* why something happens, qualitative approaches seek to *understand* the interpretations and motivations of people.

Another contrast between quantitative and qualitative research involves the sort of knowledge that researchers regard as valid. Quantitative researchers usually regard *objective* knowledge as the best form of knowing. Objectivity is the assumption that facts can and should be presented in a manner untainted by the feelings, opinions or bias of the researcher or researched. In contrast, qualitative researchers emphasise the importance of *subjective* knowledge – that which comes from a person's particular perspective. Qualitative research often involves the assumption that the sole foundation of factual knowledge is private experience, and that this private experience should be treated with seriousness.

Belief in the significance of subjective factors in qualitative research is not limited to the subjective knowledge of the researched. Qualitative analysts often assert the need for researchers to reveal the values, interests and influences associated with their own subjective experiences. This process is termed reflexivity (Hammersley and Atkinson, 1995), in that it involves researchers reflecting back on themselves and the way they conduct their research, rather than putting all their efforts into examining their research subjects. Good research involves reflexivity at several levels. First, researchers should identify the theoretical assumptions with which they are operating, along with the values and commitments to which they adhere. Second, they should reflect upon how personal biographical factors might affect the research. Finally, they should describe and reflect upon how the methods used in their research, and the context within which the research is conducted, might affect the outcome of the research.

While the commitment of quantitative research to objectivity means that it seeks to obliterate the person of the researcher from the research process, relying on verifiable methods to show the accuracy of its results, qualitative research's emphasis on reflexivity means that the subjective experiences and circumstances of the researcher come to the fore. To underline the importance of the person of the researcher, qualitative researchers often use the first person active to describe themselves in research reports, rather than the traditional, third person passive ('I noted . . .' instead of 'it was noted by the researcher . . .') (Porter, 1993a).

From what I have said above, it would seem that there is a clear divide between qualitative and quantitative research. This, I am afraid, is rather too simplistic, in that neither style of research fits neatly into these categories. The purpose of this contrast was to give as clearly as possible a flavour of the assumptions underlying these different approaches to research. In the real life of research, however, the boundaries between the approaches are far more blurred than I have described them. Thus, for example, in contradiction to what I said above about reasons and causes, my own research (Porter, 1993b) provides an example of the use of qualitative methods to uncover, if not exactly cause and effect relationships, then relationships of influence between social structures and the actions of individual nurses and doctors. You should try not to think of there being a 'right' way for qualitative research and another one for quantitative research. All of these underlying assumptions are open to question and different researchers will come to their own conclusions as to what is the most appropriate theoretical basis for their research. Indeed, a recent and welcome trend in research has been the increasing willingness of researchers to overcome these divisions through the incorporation of that which is best from both traditions into their research designs. However, while you cannot judge of piece of research by using a checklist to see if it properly subscribes to the assumptions that are supposed to underlie its approach, you can judge it on the clarity and openness with which a researcher explains the assumptions which she has adopted.

THE THEORETICAL FOUNDATIONS OF QUALITATIVE RESEARCH

Having contrasted qualitative research with quantitative research, I now wish to look more closely at the theoretical foundations of qualitative research. As with all systems of investigation, qualitative research is founded upon a number of wider assumptions, which can be classified according to four levels of understanding. These levels are termed in the rather daunting jargon of philosophy, ontology, epistemology, method-ology and methods. Before explaining what these terms mean, I should once again repeat my qualification that what is set out below is not a definitive description of what all qualitative researchers believe. Rather, it is only one (albeit common) version of the assumptions underlying the use of qualitative methods. As a result, the assumptions set out are open to debate and disagreement. They should therefore not be taken as a gospel of qualitative beliefs.

Level One: Ontology

Ontology concerns questions about what exists. In terms of its research focus, that which exists for qualitative research is the meaningful actions and interactions of individuals.

Qualitative research has been much influenced by a branch of phil-osophy known as *phenomenology*. The basic premise of phenomenology is that the nature of the outside world, independent of our thoughts about it, can never be known. All we can know is how people perceive and interpret that reality. After all, the phenomenologist asks, how do we know anything, except through the use of our senses and mental faculties? Thus for phenomenology, the aim of knowledge is not to objectively uncover the nature of the external world, but to understand how we come to know the world as we do. One of the consequences of this ontological assumption is that reality is not a single, fixed thing. It changes and develops according to people's experiences, and the social context within which they find themselves. In other words, for different people and, indeed, for the same people at different times, reality will be different. Think, for example, of going to see a film with a friend, coming out and discussing it over a coffee afterwards and discovering that your interpretations of what you saw were so different that you wondered whether you were actually in the same cinema. On a similar line, think of a film that you saw when you were young and saw again when you were older, when once again it seemed completely different from your first experience of it.

The significance of social context is crucial to our perception of reality because it is through our social interactions with others – parents, teachers, friends, health care colleagues and clients to name but a few – that our understandings and preconceptions about the nature of that reality are formed. This is not just a one-way process, since through our interactions with each other we help create the social world around us. It is for this reason that qualitative researchers often adopt the ontological position that the reality they wish to examine involves the meaningful social interaction between individuals.

As I have already noted, the ontological assumptions described above are not held by all qualitative researchers. For some, acceptance of the importance of social context implies that phenomenological understanding is not enough. They argue that the actions of individuals cannot be explained solely by the understandings and motivations of those individuals; what also needs to be taken into account are the social structures that enable and constrain the actions and interpretations of individuals (Porter, 1993b). Nevertheless, it remains true to say that phenomenology is the bedrock of most qualitative research.

The application of these ontological assumptions to nursing leads qualitative researchers to concentrate on people's experiences of being ill. As Benner and Wrubel (1989) state, 'Illness as a human experience of loss or dysfunction has a reality all its own'. Here we can see a rejection of the traditional medical model of the ontology of illness, which equates the reality of illness with physical manifestations of disease or disablement. The focus of the medical model is seen as accurate as far as it goes but too narrow, in that the reality of sickness cannot be reduced completely to biochemical processes. Proper understanding must also include the person's subjective experience of the illness, and the social context within which that experience occurs. This revision of the biomedical ontology of illness is of considerable importance, as Jerrett (1994) points out in her phenomenological study of the experiences of parents with chronically ill children: 'their subjective experience is fundamentally important not just because it involves a personal reassessment of objective reality, but because lived experience is reality'.

Level Two: Epistemology

Epistemology concerns questions about what we can know about what exists. Based on the ontological assumptions outlined above, for qualitative researchers what we can know about people's reality equates with our understanding of the meanings and motives which guide their actions and interactions.

The connection here between epistemology and ontology is clear. If the reality that qualitative researchers are concerned with consists of the experiences and understandings of people, then knowledge of reality will be knowledge of those experiences and understandings. An example of the use of this sort of epistemological assumption in nursing research is found in Melia's (1982) seminal study of student nurses. Melia argues that the reality of student nursing lay in the students' own constructions of their nursing world. As a consequence, the interest of her research 'lay in obtaining the student nurses' view of nursing, in other words to allow the students to "tell it as it is"'.

For Melia, 'telling it as it is' meant gaining knowledge of the experiences and understandings of the nurses that she was researching. However, gaining such knowledge is not a simple matter. The problem is that it is not possible to get inside people's minds in order to fully understand their experiences. For one thing, those experiences will always be filtered through the understandings of the researcher, and it is very difficult to tell the degree of distortion that this entails. As Melia (1982) notes, the role of the qualitative researcher in the production of data is crucial. Because of these problems, the epistemological claims of qualitative research are cautious. Qualitative researchers accept that absolute knowledge of other people's reality is not possible, and our knowledge of that reality will always be an approximation that will be affected by the interpretations of the researcher (Porter, 1993a).

Level Three: Methodology

Methodology concerns questions about the manner in which we can gain knowledge about what exists. Qualitative researchers argue that reality can be discovered by looking at it through the perspective of the individuals living in it.

Qualitative researchers are required to interpret as accurately as possible the experiences, meanings and motives of subjects, from the perspectives of those subjects. This will largely depend upon the researcher's knowledge of and familiarity with the social setting being studied. Gaining this familiarity requires a considerable period of time, in which the researcher immerses herself as fully as possible in the lives or work of the people she is studying.

However, irrespective of the degree of immersion, the influence of the researcher's own perspective will remain, so it is necessary to adopt a methodology which can take account of this. Here we return to reflexivity. By openly examining and reporting how her own experiences and understandings have affected the nature of research, the researcher displays her influence upon the research to readers, who can then make up their own minds about persuasiveness of the findings.

Once again, we can see this process in the work of Melia (1982), where she gives a reflexive account of her research, outlining for the reader the amount of knowledge she had of the social world of the student nurses in her study. She points out that, having trained and practised as a nurse, she was reasonably familiar with the working world of student nurses. However, she is careful to point out gaps in her experience. Most significantly, she notes that her experience of training was not the three-year apprenticeship programme in which her subjects were studying, and that she had trained in a different institution to that in her study.

Melia's reflexive account gives readers the opportunity to judge for themselves her knowledge of, and familiarity with the world of her research subjects, and thus to assess better the accuracy of her reproduction of their perspectives. Without the sort of statistical tests for reliability and validity to which quantitative researchers can avail themselves, the kind of reflexivity displayed by Melia is crucial for qualitative research if it is to be persuasive.

Level Four: Methods

Methods are the techniques used to collect evidence about what exists. The methods used by qualitative researchers can be divided into two broad approaches. The first approach is designed to enable researchers to become involved in the social world of the subjects they are studying, in order to gain direct experience of their understandings, meanings and motives which provide the basis for their actions and interactions. This approach is epitomised by the method of participant observation. The second approach is designed to give research subjects the opportunity to describe and explain, in their own words, their understandings, meanings and motives which provide the basis for their actions and interactions. The most common method here is that of in-depth interviewing.

IN-DEPTH INTERVIEWS

In-depth interviewing is probably the most common qualitative method used in nursing research. Other terms that you may come across for describing this method are 'unstructured interviewing' (if there is no prior format for the interview), 'semi-structured interviewing' (if there is some format, but the interview is allowed to go in directions that are beyond the bounds of that format), 'informal' or 'ethnographic interviewing'. The point of in-depth interviewing is to give subjects the opportunity to describe their experiences and understandings in their own words.

In-depth interviewing can either be used on its own or in combination with participant observation. When combined with participant observation, the information supplied by interviewees can help explain and contextualise the actions and interactions seen by the researcher during the observation component of the research.

Rather than knowing precisely all the questions that she will ask beforehand, the qualitative researcher comes to the in-depth interview with only a general plan about the direction which the conversation will take. There are two main reasons why qualitative researchers tend to avoid questionnaires or heavily structured interview formats. First, it is contended that because informal interviews provide interviewees with a situation more akin to natural conversation, where they can talk freely about their lives in a non-threatening environment, they will tend to be more forthcoming. Second, it is argued that the rather inflexible construction of questions in structured interviews and questionnaires means that there is a danger that the line of questioning will simply reinforce the questioner's assumptions about the nature of the problem she is examining. This leads to two problems. First, interviewees may feel pressurised into giving what they perceive as the 'right' answer, i.e. the answer that they think the interviewer wants them to give. Second, there is a danger that the researcher will go down the wrong track, asking inappropriate questions about the problem they are investigating. If interviewees do not have the opportunity to contribute to the research beyond the confines of a pre-determined structure, then such errors may go unnoticed by the researcher. There is less danger of these problems occurring in in-depth interviews because they allow the interviewee to have more influence over the content and direction of the interview.

There are many examples of in-depth interviewing in nursing research. One is Wuest's and Stern's (1991) study of families of children with persistent middle ear problems, designed to identify the factors that most influenced family interaction in such circumstances. Wuest and Stern discovered that one of the main concerns of family members was management of the day-to-day practicalities of family life. Through their interviews, they discovered that parents felt that they were not getting adequate support from health professionals to help them cope with their situation. Wuest and Stern concluded that nurses have the potential to greatly help families with chronically ill children by providing this service.

Oral History

A special type of the in-depth interview, known as oral history, is used if the social setting that the researcher wants to find out about existed in the past. As in in-depth interviews, interviewees in oral histories are given the opportunity to describe and explain their past experiences in their own words.

A good example of the use of this method in nursing research is Keddy et al.'s (1986) examination of the relationship between nurses and doctors in Canada in the 1920s and 1930s. In order to find out about what it was like to be a nurse at that time, Keddy et al. taped 34 semi-structured interviews with older nurses, asking them to recount events and experiences from their nursing past. One of the main themes that emerged from the interviews was the importance of the relationship between nurses and doctors at the time, a relationship in which doctors enjoyed almost complete authority, where they had control over the hiring, firing and education of nurses. However, Keddy et al. were not only interested in the arrangements that pertained; they also wanted to find out what the nurses felt about those arrangements as they experienced them. Unsurprisingly, frustration was one of the more common experiences expressed.

Focus Groups

This qualitative method takes the form of group interviewing, in which members of the group are encouraged to discuss the issues at hand amongst themselves, as well as with the researcher. What makes focus groups unique as a form of interviewing is that they make use of the interactions within the group to gain data that would not be so easily accessible in one-to-one interviews (Morgan, 1988). Discussing issues with peers can help people to clarify their ideas to a greater degree than would be the case if they were being interviewed on their own. In a way focus groups lie somewhere between in-depth interviewing and participant observation, in that while they are a form of group interview, the researcher also has the opportunity to observe the dynamics of group interaction, albeit in an artificial setting. An example of the use of focus groups in health care research is Morgan's and Spanish's (1985) study of how middle-aged men think of heart attacks.

PARTICIPANT OBSERVATION

Participant observation is the classic qualitative method. Its name provides a good description of what it involves – in this method researchers participate in the daily life of their research subjects, while simultaneously observing the actions and interpretations of those subjects while they go about their day-to-day business. The aim is to gain an 'insider's' view of the group under study. This is attained both by the researcher's direct experience of what it is like to live or work in the social circumstances under examination, and by the information provided to the researcher by members of the group under study while they go about their everyday activities.

Data gathered through participant observation may be recorded electronically through audio or video taping. However, the most common method of recording is to write down observations and thoughts in the form of what are termed 'fieldnotes'. These are detailed descriptions of social situations and interactions that occur in the 'field' of research – field being the term used for the location where data are gathered.

Participant observation goes back a long way. For example, the writings of Marco Polo could be described as belonging to this genre. However, it was not until the early twentieth century that it was developed from the rather unsystematic format of travellers' tales into a more scientific method of enquiry. This development was pioneered by European anthropologists such as Malinowski (1922), who used it to study non-western cultures, and by the 'Chicago School' of sociology, who used it to examine western subcultures.

Despite being a well established and popular method of research in both anthropology and sociology, there are limitations to its use in nursing research, especially when the proposed subjects of research are health care clients. There are good practical reasons for this – it is difficult for a healthy researcher to participate in the social world of those who are ill. Given that much qualitative nursing research focuses upon this group, the possibilities of participant observation are somewhat limited. However, those suffering from illness are not the only group of interest to qualitative nursing researchers. There is also much useful information to be gained by examining how and why nurses go about their work in the way that they do, and it is perfectly possible for nursing researchers to participate in the social world of clinical nurses. One example of this approach is my own work into the influence of gender upon nurses' professional relationships with medical colleagues (Porter, 1992). The findings of this study were based on three months of participant observation as a staff nurse in an intensive care unit. As a integral member of the nursing staff of the unit, I was able to immerse myself in the occupational lives of my colleagues.

The aim of my research was to discover the nature of nurse–doctor interactions, to see how gender affected those interactions, and to find out how nurses experienced, felt about and interpreted them. First, I looked to see if there were any differences in the quality of interaction based on the sex of those involved. I discovered that while the gender of a nurse had little effect upon the quality of interaction between nurse and doctor, the gender of a doctor did. I found that female doctors were often less authoritarian in their dealings with nurses than male doctors. In looking at how nurses interpreted gender issues as they related to their interactions with doctors, I discovered that they resented doctors' expectations for them to act as handmaidens, and felt perfectly willing to respond to medical arrogance by being assertive. However, while nurses were prepared to criticise doctors who were openly chauvinistic, they did not see this as a problem that related to the occupation of medicine as a whole. Rather than seeing sexism as an integral part of the nurse–doctor relationship, they regarded it as an individual issue concerning those male doctors who were most openly arrogant in their dealings with female nurses.

The point of this brief description of my research is to show how participant observation can be used both to discover the nature of interaction in a social setting, and to illuminate the understandings and motives of those involved in the interactions.

CONVERSATION ANALYSIS

Conversation analysis is considerably different in its approach from the methods examined thus far, in that it uses more formal, scientific procedures to gain and analyse data. The aim of conversation analysis is to study *how* people talk to each other in everyday settings. In other words, the emphasis is more on the form of interaction, rather than its content. Conversation analysis attempts to uncover how people technically construct their conversations so as to accomplish ordered conversational interaction. Because even the smallest nuances in conversations are important in this type of research, the use of a tape recorder is essential. Even better is a video recorder, in that it can give giving a fuller picture of the processes of communication by recording gestures and facial expressions.

In conversation analysis, the researcher takes on a passive role, allowing research subjects to engage in day-to-day conversational activities, recording them while they do so. These recordings are then transcribed using specialised annotation in which, for example, pauses, interruptions and overlaps of speech are marked. Conversation is transcribed phonetically, rather than translated into standard English. You may wonder what is the point of this qualitative method. Conversation analysts argue that it is important because talk is the building block of all social interaction, and conversely, that broader social processes are manifested in conversational interaction.

A good example of how conversation analysis can add to health care knowledge is to be found in Brewer et al.'s (1991) study of the conversations of children with severe learning difficulties. Through close study of their conversations, Brewer et al. discovered that, contrary to popular assumptions that children with learning difficulties are communicatively incompetent, these children possessed considerable conversational skills. One child, especially, was seen as highly adept at orchestrating interactions with others. However, the other children were far from being incompetent conversationalists, being capable of appropriate response and turn-taking. By methodically analysing the conversation of children with severe learning difficulties into its basic component parts, Brewer et al. demonstrated the high degree to which their conversations were organised, thus providing a useful challenge to preconceptions about the communicative competence of children with learning disabilities.

GROUNDED THEORY

Grounded theory is not simply another method of doing qualitative research; it is far more than that, in that it provides its own methodological basis for the conduct of research. Once again, this points us to the fact that in qualitative research there is no one correct way of doing things, but many competing models. It will be remembered that qualitative researchers are concerned about not imposing their own ideas and assumptions on the research, but allowing research subjects to express their understandings on their own terms. Grounded theory takes this injunction very seriously indeed, and as a result proposes that qualitative research should be conducted in a purely *inductive* fashion.

Here we need to understand the difference between inductive and hypothetico–deductive logics. Hypothetico–deductive explanation is the form of logic normally used in science. Here the researcher starts out with a hypothesis (a general proposition about the nature of the subject matter to be examined), and then proceeds to draw out (or deduce) from that hypothesis what would happen if the hypothesis is correct. The final stage of this approach is to examine the subject matter to see if the predictions deduced from the hypothesis actually occur. The hypothesis is regarded as at least provisionally confirmed if successful predictions have been made. The core of this method is that it starts with general statements and then uses specific instances to confirm or deny the veracity of those general statements. Induction starts at precisely the opposite end, at which examination of particular instances are the starting point. General statements emerge (or are induced) from the patterns of specific instances observed, rather than being posited at the beginning of the research process.

In grounded theory, the aim is not simply to avoid hypotheses, but to avoid any sort of preconceptions about the nature of the group under study (Glaser and Strauss, 1967). Instead, the researcher's knowledge of the field of study should come solely from information gained in the field. The grounded theory researcher starts not with a literature review, but directly with participant observation (although other qualitative methods may also be used). Data gathered in this way are then sorted (or coded) into various categories or themes. The relationship between these categories is examined, and the linkages that are made lead the researcher to develop what is termed in the grounded theory jargon, 'core categories', which are similar to the hypotheses of deductive research, bar the fact that they have emerged from examination of the data, rather than being posited before the data have been gathered.

Grounded theory is a popular approach within qualitative nursing research (see, for example, Wilde et al., 1993). One reason for this is that many aspects of nursing are under-researched. This means that the researcher has very little previous material to go on. It therefore makes sense to start from scratch, accepting no assumptions as to the reasons behind the actions and interactions of the group under study. The development of theory from data that have been gathered from real settings helps ensure the appropriateness of the theory. However, some argue that, in many cases, grounded theory takes induction too far. This is specifically the case in areas where research has previously been done. In avoiding the use of previous research literature so as to circumvent the problem of entering the field with presuppositions, grounded theory researchers may be in danger of re-inventing the wheel. In other words, previous literature is there to be used, without allowing it to predetermine the outcome of the research (Porter, 1996). As a result, many qualitative researchers adopt a less strictly inductive method than that promoted by grounded theory.

THE AIM OF QUALITATIVE RESEARCH IN NURSING

From our examination of qualitative research, we can see how its purpose is to describe and understand the meanings and motives that lie behind the actions and interactions of identified groups of people. The focus of qualitative research in nursing may be on patients, as in Johnson's (1994) study of the way in which overweight people restructure their perspectives during the process of dieting; on relatives, as in Jerrett's (1994) study of parents with chronically ill children; or it can be on nurses themselves, as in Melia's (1982) study of the lives of student nurses.

This is not to say that qualitative research is confined to the description of the understandings and interactions of particular groups; it can also be used to test more general theories about the nature of the social world as pertaining to health and health care. An example of this broader, more theoretical approach can be found in May's (1992) qualitative analysis of the degree to which Foucault's (1973) notion of the 'clinical gaze', which asserts that the relationship between doctors and patients is one of medical surveillance, can be applied to the nurse-patient relationship.

Qualitative research can also be useful in policy evaluation. An example of this approach is Mason's (1994) comparative study of the contrasting perspectives of officialdom and mothers in relation to community maternal and child health policies in Jamaica and the north of Ireland.

THE IMPORTANCE OF QUALITATIVE RESEARCH IN NURSING

Over the last two decades, qualitative research has become an increasingly popular and influential approach within nursing research, and there are good reasons to believe that its influence will continue to grow. These reasons relate to changes in the focus of nursing care. Most notable is the change in nursing philosophy away from a task-centred approach to patients, towards a more holistic perspective towards care, which emphasises the importance of the experience of illness and the wants, needs and fears that such experience engenders in different people in different ways. This change in the focus of nursing practice has inevitably led to a change in focus of the sort of knowledge that nurses require. This in turn means that nursing researchers are required, at least in part, to adopt research methodologies which are designed to gain knowledge about the experiences of illness and care. This is where qualitative research comes into its own.

REFERENCES

Benner, P. and Wrubel, J. (1989) *The Primacy of Caring*. Menlo Park, CA: Addison-Wesley.

Brewer, J.D., McBride, G., and Yearley, S. (1991) Orchestrating an encounter: a note on the talk of mentally handicapped children, *Sociology of Health and Illness*, 13, 58–67.

Foucault, M. (1973) *The Birth of the Clinic*. London: Tavistock.

Glaser, B. and Strauss, A. (1967) *The Discovery of Grounded Theory*. New York: Aldine.

Hammersley, M. and Atkinson, P. (1995) *Ethnography: Principles in Practice*, 2nd edn. London: Routledge.

Jerrett, M. (1994) Parents' experience of coming to know the care of a chronically ill child, *Journal of Advanced Nursing*, 19, 1050–6.

Johnson, R. (1994) Restructuring: an emerging theory on the process of losing weight, in: J.P. Smith (ed.), *Models, Theories and Concepts*. Oxford: Blackwell: 31–46.

Keddy, B., Jones Gillis, M., Jacobs, P., Burton, H., and Rogers, M. (1986) The doctor-nurse relationship: an historical perspective, *Journal of Advanced Nursing*, 7, 327–35.

Malinowski, E. (1922) *Argonauts of the Western Pacific*. New York: Dutton.

Mason, C. (1994) Maternal and child health needs in Northern Ireland and Jamaica: official and lay perspectives, *Qualitative Health Research*, 4, 74–93.

May, C. (1992) Individual care? Power and subjectivity in therapeutic relationships. *Sociology*, 26, 589–602.

Melia, K. (1982) 'Tell it as it is' – qualitative methodology and nursing research: understanding the student nurse's world, *Journal of Advanced Nursing*, 7, 327–35.

Morgan, D. (1988) *Focus Groups as Qualitative Research*. London: Sage.

Morgan, D. and Spanish, M. (1985) Social interaction and the cognitive organisation of health-relevant behaviour, *Sociology of Health and Illness*, 7, 401–22.

Porter, S. (1992) Women in a women's job: the gendered experience of nurses, *Sociology of Health and Illness*, 14, 510–27.

Porter, S. (1993a) Nursing research conventions: objectivity or obfuscation? *Journal of Advanced Nursing*, 18, 137–43.

Porter, S. (1993b) Critical realist ethnography: the case of racism and professionalism in a medical setting, *Sociology*, 27, 591–609.

Porter, S. (1996) Qualitative analysis, in D. Cormack (ed.), *The Research Process in Nursing*, 3rd edn. Oxford: Blackwell: 330–40.

Wilde, B., Starrin, B., Larsson, G., and Larsson, M. (1993) Quality of care from a patient's perspective: a grounded theory study, *Scandinavian Journal of Caring Sciences*, 7, 113–20.

Wuest, J. and Stern, P. (1991) Empowerment and primary health care: the challenge for nurses, *Qualitative Health Research*, 1, 80–99.

4

Quantitative Research

Roger Watson

INTRODUCTION

Quantitative research methods are widely applicable in nursing research. In order to understand quantitative methods it is essential to understand the concept of measurement and the parameters by which measurement may be judged

Background to Quantitative Methods

Quantitative methods are derived from the natural sciences. In chemistry, quantities of substances have to be measured accurately and all the phenomena of physics such as light, heat and electricity are expressed in measurements (Jardine, 1964). Likewise, in the biological sciences, measurement is important. In order to gauge the activity of an enzyme in a tissue it has to be compared against measured amounts of the enzyme. Measurement is important in the application of the natural sciences, for example, in the preparation of compounds such as drugs and in engineering.

It is also from the natural sciences that quantitative research designs are derived. The classic research method in the natural sciences is experimentation whereby conditions are manipulated in order to test the possibility of a proposed outcome. However, there is also analytical research which is concerned with analysing the constituent parts of substances. In both cases there are analogous research methods which are applicable to nursing research.

Nursing Research

Nursing research falls mainly within the realm of the social sciences and is described as an 'umbrella term for all research into nursing practice and issues related to it' (Parahoo, 1997: 7). As such the quantitative and the qualitative research methods of psychology and sociology have been successfully adopted and adapted into nursing research. The expression 'nursing research' will be used throughout this chapter to indicate research into nursing which falls within the domain of the social sciences.

MEASUREMENT

Measurement has synonyms including 'assessment', 'estimation' and 'determination' according to a thesaurus (Seaton et al., 1986). These convey a sense of attempting to gauge the amount of something or to compare amounts. We are familiar with measuring amounts of substances, for instance in cooking and lengths of time and, as nurses, vital signs such as pulse and temperature. However, is it possible to measure more abstract concepts such as happiness or sadness? In nursing research we are often concerned with measuring such abstract concepts and we should have a grasp of the levels at which measurement may be made in order to understand how different types of measurement compare.

Levels of Measurement

Measurement may be made at four levels: nominal, ordinal, interval and ratio and these will be compared and contrasted below. Levels of measurement run from the lowest to the highest as listed above with nominal being the lowest level of measurement and ratio being the highest level (Walsh, 1990).

Nominal level

This lowest level of measurement is hardly measurement at all and is really concerned with classifying objects or people in order that they may be distinguished from one another and, concomitantly, grouped together where possible (Walsh, 1990). However, calling this the lowest level of measurement should not mislead the reader into thinking that it is neither important nor useful.

An example from nursing where nominal level measurement may be used is in the classification of a group of patients according to their diagnosis or according to the ward in which they are staying. For example, patients with a myocardial infarction could be labelled '1' and patients with emphysema could be labelled '2' and so on, or the numbers could be ascribed to patients staying on Ward A and Ward B respectively. Note that, despite the fact numbers have been ascribed to the patients, they have no value as such and are merely a way of distinguishing, on the one hand, and grouping, on the other. There is a weakness in nominal measurement: the categories into which patients are placed may not be quite discrete. For example, whereas the ward on which a patient is staying is quite discrete (unless the patient changes wards), what number would be ascribed to a patient with a myocardial infarction and emphysema? It is quite possible that a third category would have to be used.

Ordinal level

Ordinal level measurements are used to place objects or people relative to one another and, in this sense, are superior to nominal measurements which merely classify (Walsh, 1990). This is only a limited form of measurement; nevertheless it has found wide application in nursing research and, as will be explained later, can be used to generate higher levels of measurement. As an example, if nurses were trying to compare the recovery of a group of patients from a procedure but there was no established scale with which to do this then an ordinal measure could be used. One way in which they could do this would be to classify the patients relative to one another as 'not recovered', 'slightly recovered', 'almost recovered' and 'recovered' and to assign numbers 1–4 to each of these measures. In this way they would be making a very crude measure on the patients. The cardinal feature of this system of measurement is that the numbers, while signifying relative measures, do not have any absolute value as such. For instance, using the example above, a patient who is described as 'recovered' (4) is not twice as recovered as a patient who is 'slightly recovered' (2). Therefore, the numbers have a limited use in themselves but there are statistical tests, to be described later, which can be used with ordinal numbers.

Interval level

Interval level measurements are more familiar to us and an excellent example from the natural sciences is the measurement of temperature using the Celsius (°C) scale. An example from the social sciences is the measurement of intelligence (IQ). In both of these examples there is an equal distance, or interval, between successive units of measurement (Walsh, 1990). For example, there is an equal change in temperature between 10°C and 11°C to that between 15°C and 16°C. Similarly, differences between successive points on an IQ scale are equal. However, in both of the above examples the scales do not have a true point of origin, i.e. a zero point, therefore there is a limit to the use of interval level measurements. This can best be expressed by saying that someone with an IQ of 70 is not half as intelligent as someone with an IQ of 140; nor is a temperature of 40°C twice as warm as a temperature of 20°C. Despite the equal intervals between measurements, interval level measurements are arbitrary and used both for convenience, as in the case of temperature and also in the absence of a direct measurement, as in the case of intelligence. It should be noted that interval level measurements are usually the highest level of measurement attainable in nursing research.

Ratio level

Ratio level measurements have all the properties of the above measurements in that they can classify objects, place them relative to one another and provide an equal interval measure (Walsh, 1990). However, they also have a true point of origin, a zero point, and these are the highest level of measurement. Again, we are familiar with many examples such as time and distance; clearly, two hours are twice as long as one hour and ten kilometres are twice as long as five kilometres. Despite their utility and predominance in the natural sciences, it is unusual to be able to make ratio level measurements in nursing research.

QUANTITATIVE RESEARCH DESIGNS

In the natural sciences, as indicated above, particular research designs are employed: experimental and analytical. These both find counterparts in nursing research and these will be considered in this section. In nursing research these designs are referred to as experimental and correlational, respectively (Bryman and Cramer, 1997). The latter is sometimes referred to as survey or descriptive research. Before proceeding, the concepts of variables and the concept of the hypothesis should be considered.

Variables

In terms of quantitative research designs a variable is anything that can be measured or manipulated in order to fulfil the criteria of the research. For example, time may be a variable either as an outcome of a research design – time taken to complete a task, or as a parameter of the design if individuals are given different lengths of time to complete a task and the outcome of that task subsequently evaluated. Likewise, a measure of patient satisfaction with a stay in hospital or the extent of recovery after a fixed number of days may also be variables.

Dependent and independent variables

In some cases variables may directly manipulated, i.e. under the control of the researcher such as a length of treatment or may only, potentially, be indirectly manipulated by changing the parameters of the research, such as level of pain after different lengths of treatment. This leads to the concepts of dependence and independence of variables, which apply to both experimental and correlational research.

An independent variable is one which is not, for the purposes of a particular piece of research, influenced by the variables which are dependent upon it (Walsh, 1990). In the case of experimental research, the independent variable is the one which is manipulated by the researcher, for example, the administration of a treatment. On the other hand, a dependent variable is one which is dependent upon an independent variable, and, using the same example, the effect of the treatment such as level of pain, would be the dependent variable (Walsh, 1990). The researcher cannot directly manipulate the dependent variable except by administering the treatment – assuming that there is some link between the treatment and the level of pain. In correlational research it is not always entirely clear which variables are dependent and which are independent and this will be considered in the relevant section below.

Experimental Designs

In an experiment the researcher is able to set up the conditions under which the research will take place (Polit and Hungler, 1995). The most 'scientific' version of the experiment, involving human subjects, is the clinical trial which is employed widely in medicine in the testing of new drugs but has found some application in nursing (Watson and Kuhn, 1990). The first essential requirement of the clinical trial is that there are at least two groups of patients, one which receives a treatment and one which does not. The former is referred to as the 'experimental' group and the latter is referred to as the 'control' group (Polit and Hungler, 1995). The effectiveness of the treatment is then evaluated based on measuring and comparing some parameter in both groups. The second essential requirement of the clinical trial is that the patients involved in the clinical trial are randomly assigned to either the experimental or the control group (Polit and Hungler, 1995). Random allocation minimises any bias which the researcher may have, referred to as systematic bias, or any other unseen factors which may influence the outcome of the clinical trial. Randomisation will be explained below.

There are several variations on the theme of the experiment where the design described above is relaxed and these are referred to as quasi-experiments. This may be required where, for either ethical or practical reasons, it is not possible to allocate at random (Parahoo, 1997). For example, it may be possible to administer a new drug only in one particular hospital, therefore all the patients in the experimental group come from one hospital and all the controls come from another. It can be seen that this would lead to problems in interpreting the trial. Any difference between the experimental and control group may be the result of differences in the hospitals and not in the administration of the new drug.

Correlational Designs

Correlational designs do not involve any manipulation of variables or the setting up of groups for comparative purposes as in experimental designs. Rather, they use a sub-group of people from the population, known as a sample, and measure variables of interest within that group. For example, if a nurse administrator wished to investigate what factors were related to the length of time for which patients remained in hospital then this could be accomplished using a correlational design. Clearly, an experimental design would be inappropriate because it would not be possible, in advance, to set up groups based on the length of time for which they remained in hospital.

Instead of one outcome by which groups of people are compared, in correlational designs the researcher can measure a range of variables and then investigate relationships amongst them. In the above example the nurse administrator might choose, in addition to length of stay, to measure social class, income, number of people living at home, occupation and even satisfaction with the stay in hospital. After the data have been gathered it is possible to analyse them in order to see if length of stay is related to any of these parameters. Obviously, it may not be related to any of them; correlational research is really only as good as the variables which are selected for measurement.

As mentioned above, a note of caution about interpreting correlational research studies should be issued. It is not always possible to identify, in a relationship between two variables, which is the independent variable and which is the dependent variable. In other words, which variable is the 'cause' and which is the 'effect' (Polit and Hungler, 1997). In fact, any relationship between two variables may be secondary or even spurious. For instance, if it was found in a social survey that there was a relationship between intelligence (measured using IQ) and social class then it cannot be assumed that being in a low social class leads to lower intelligence. It could equally be the case that having a lower intelligence leads a person to remain in a lower social class. Furthermore, it cannot be assumed that there is any direct cause and effect relationship between the two variables; both may be the result of some other factor, such as genetic predisposition, which has not been measured.

Randomisation

Randomisation was mentioned above in relation to allocating patients to groups in a clinical trial. However, randomisation also applies to correlational studies. The purpose behind randomisation is to minimise any bias which may take place in the selection of subjects for research and which may, thereby, bias the results of the research. It also allows the results of the research to be applied to the general population. There are two types of bias: one is systematic bias (Polit and Hungler, 1995) and the other is random bias. Systematic bias will arise if the researcher assigns people to groups in a clinical trial or selects them for inclusion in a survey according to certain attributes which will influence the outcome of the study. Clearly, there need to be criteria whereby subjects, i.e. people involved in the research, become eligible for inclusion in a study, for example having a specific diagnosis or being within a certain age range. Thereafter, the selection or assignment should be random. Imagine, for instance, a clinical trial where the effect of a novel nursing care procedure on recovery from a surgical procedure was being investigated. If the researcher chose to put all the younger patients in the group receiving the new procedure and all the older ones in the control group, the results of the research would certainly be biased in favour of the treatment group.

Random bias occurs owing to natural differences between individuals. It cannot be controlled or eliminated; it can be minimised by randomisation. Randomisation merely ensures that all individuals who are eligible to be included in a study have an equal chance of being selected or assigned to a particular group.

There are many ways of introducing randomness into a study such as drawing names out of a hat or employing computers. A standard method is the use of random number tables whereby eligible individuals are assigned a number and then random number tables consulted by starting at a particular point in the table and moving in one direction until the allocated numbers appear (Atkinson, 1996). On this basis individuals can be either recruited into a survey or allocated to a group in a clinical trial.

Despite the importance of randomisation it is often not possible to employ it in a study for a variety of reasons. As described above, in a clinical trial it may not be possible randomly to assign patient to treatment and control groups in which case the trial becomes quasi-experimental. In survey research it is often inconvenient to make a random selection and it is the case that subjects are obtained in a systematic fashion or on a convenience basis (Polit and Hungler, 1995). The researcher who has, for whatever reason, relaxed the parameters of a study by omitting randomisation should always report this in the results of the study. This information is essential to the reader as this will let the reader know how possible it is to generalise from the study. The results of a survey in which subjects are not selected on a random basis are not, strictly speaking, applicable to the general population.

Sampling

All quantitative research is concerned with generating new knowledge applicable to the general population, i.e. to all the people who could possibly be involved in a study. The only way to ensure that the outcome of a study is applicable to the population is to include in the study all the people who are eligible to be in the study. However, this is impractical and, with the possible exception of a national census, is rarely achieved. The standard procedure for any type of research – quantitative or qualitative – is to conduct the research on a sub-section of the population, in other words on a sample (Atkinson, 1996). The concept of randomisation applies to sampling in order that results may be applied to the population and this has been discussed above. However, this is only one aspect of sampling. The other important aspect of sampling is how large a sample should be and there is no easy answer to this question. It is beyond the scope of this chapter to consider sampling in any detail but it is possible to provide some direction.

The objective of sampling is to ensure that a sample is truly representative of the population from which the sample is taken but also to remain practical in terms of the research. On the one hand, therefore, the sample needs to be sufficiently large (clearly, one person would not be representative of the population) but not so large that it becomes too expensive or unwieldy for a research project. Ultimately the answer to the sample size rests on what the researcher intends to do with the results in terms of analyses and this is related to the statistical tests which will, ultimately, be employed. Tables and mathematical formulae are available (Cohen, 1992; Polit and Hungler, 1995) but, as a rule of thumb, in nursing research using questionnaires, it is reasonable to expect that there should be between five and ten subjects per question (Kline, 1994). Questionnaires, as described below, are the most commonly applied method of gathering quantitative data in nursing research.

Another reason for ensuring that sample size is adequate may be demonstrated by referring to experimental research where differences between groups are investigated. If the number of subjects in each group is not large enough then the researcher cannot be sure, in the event that no difference between groups is observed following administration of a treatment, that any real difference is not being masked by random variation in the subjects. If sample size is adequate then the experiment is said to have sufficient statistical power (Polit and Hungler, 1995). Failure to address the issue of power, through ensuring adequate sample size leads to Type II error whereby a real difference between groups (or a real relationship between variables in the case of correlational research) is not observed (Walsh, 1990).

RESEARCH QUESTIONS AND HYPOTHESES

Knowledge may be developed through research either by testing theories or developing them. This is not the place to give a detailed consideration of the relationship between theory and knowledge. However, it is appropriate to consider how research may contribute to the process of theory development. Theories tend to be very abstract notions of how the world is organised. For the purposes of research the ideas contained in a theory require to be expressed in such a way that they may be investigated practically – they must be operationalised (Bryman and Cramer, 1997). The first part of this process is to develop a research question, the purpose of which is to guide the research that will be carried out. For example, if we theorise that females in nursing view caring differently from males in nursing then an obvious research question is, simply, 'do females in nursing view caring differently from males in nursing?'

In order to answer this research question, further operationalisation is required and this will involve finding some way of measuring caring and, subsequently, developing a specific hypothesis which can be tested by means of the research and subsequent analysis. Assuming that aspects of caring among nurses can be measured then our hypothesis would be that female nurses would score differently on these measures from male nurses. Having formulated a hypothesis and gathered the necessary data the next step is to establish whether the data are confirming the hypothesis or not and the means by which a hypothesis may be tested will be considered below. If our hypothesis that female nurses score differently on the measure of caring from male nurses is upheld, then we have evidence that the answer to our research question is positive and that our theory is correct. However, while we have support for our theory, we have not proved it as such (Jardine, 1964) and we should always be aware that an alternative approach, possibly using a different measure of caring, might produce conflicting results.

QUESTIONNAIRES

Questionnaires are the means by which the majority of nursing research is carried out and questionnaire development is a subject worthy of a chapter in its own right. Questionnaires need to be relatively simple, readable and relevant to the research question (Sheatsley, 1983). This section is concerned with the use of questionnaires as measurement tools in nursing research. In order for a questionnaire to have utility in quantitative research it needs to generate a measurement which is expressed as a number. The meaning which can be ascribed to that number will be considered below; this section will be confined to the generation of numbers from questionnaires.

The standard way in which numbers are generated from questionnaires is to provide a set of responses or a range within which a response may be made to a series of simple questions. For example, in a questionnaire about caring a nurse could be asked to rate a response to a series of questions of the type 'do you consider listening to a patient to be caring?' and the response would be 'yes', 'no' or 'don't know'. Alternatively you could ask the nurse to rate agreement with the statement 'listening to a patient constitutes caring' and the response could be given on a five point scale running from 'strongly agree' at one end to 'strongly disagree' at the other (Watson and Lea, 1997). This is known as a Likert scale (Polit and Hungler, 1995). Finally, instead of asking the nurse to indicate agreement as described above you could provide a range of very definite statements such as 'I strongly agree that listening to a patient constitutes caring', 'I agree that listening to a patient constitutes caring' and so on, asking the nurse to ring the appropriate response. There are psychometric arguments for and against all of the above styles of producing question-naires but, in common, they have the ability to be scored. Usually, with Likert scale type questionnaires the scores for a series of questions are summed and an overall score for the questionnaire is produced.

A question arises about which level of measurement the scores from questionnaires, derived as described above, represent. Clearly, the indi-vidual responses to questions are ordinal and it is normally the summed responses which are used for research but it is normal to treat the individual responses as interval measures (Ferguson and Cox, 1993). The importance of this assumption is that the possibility of applying a range of statistical tests, known as parametric tests, exists rather than being able to apply a limited range of non-parametric tests. The real distinction between data to which these two sets of tests may be applied is whether or not the results from such questionnaires are normally distributed. The concept of the normal distribution need not detain us long here but suffice to say that, provided the number of people responding to the ques-tionnaire is sufficiently large then it is safe to assume, and subsequently treat, the data as being interval level. Thereby, they are suitable for the application of parametric statistical tests (Bryman and Cramer, 1997).

Reliability and Validity

A questionnaire is not an end in itself but a means to an end: producing a score which represents a measure of the phenomenon in which we are interested for the purposes of our research. However, we cannot assume that a measure generated by a questionnaire necessarily measures what we are interested in and there are two very important parameters: reliability and validity, which should be understood in relation to questionnaires. Briefly, reliability is the extent to which a measure is able to measure the same phenomenon consistently and validity is the extent to which a measure actually measures the phenomenon we are interested in (Bowling, 1995). It should be noted that it is possible to have a reliable measure which is not valid but it is not possible to have a valid measure which is not reliable. In other words, validity is predicated upon reliability.

In order to understand this further, consider the use of a ruler to make measurements of length. If the ruler is standard, in other words, the units (e.g. centimetres) conform to an agreed standard, then measurements made with the ruler will be both reliable and valid. Imagine, however, if the ruler has units marked on it which are not standard, for example each unit is called a centimetre but is only 0.75 of a centimetre, then the ruler would be capable of making reliable, i.e. consistent, measures but these would not be valid.

In the case of a ruler it is possible to check its reliability by comparing the unit measurements with a standard measure. However, in the case of a questionnaire this is not as simple. Nevertheless, there is an established test for checking the internal consistency of a questionnaire called Cronbach's alpha (Bryman and Cramer, 1997). Cronbach's alpha lies between zero and one. This test, the details of which are beyond the scope of this chapter, checks the extent to which each of the items (i.e. individual questions) is measuring the same phenomenon. If some items in the questionnaire are not making reliable measures of the phenomenon of interest then this is indicated by a low Cronbach's alpha score and these items may then be eliminated from the questionnaire. An adequate level of Cronbach's alpha is greater than 0.80. Therefore, the reliability of a questionnaire can be relatively easily addressed. On the other hand, validity is less easy to establish.

The first step in determining the validity of a questionnaire is to establish that it is reliable. Nevertheless, some steps towards ensuring validity may be taken during the development of the questionnaire and this involves ensuring that the questionnaire has content and face validity. Content validity, while efforts have been made to quantify this (Lynn, 1986), essentially involves looking at each item in the questionnaire and ensuring that it is related to the phenomenon of interest (Bowling, 1995). This can be achieved by using questions which are based on concepts derived from literature related to the phenomenon of interest and also deriving new questions and asking experts in the area of interest to look at the questions. Face validity is more nebulous but, essentially, means the extent to which the questionnaire looks sensible to those individuals who will be responding to it (Bowling, 1995).

There are more complex aspects of validity and these include criterion and concurrent validity whereby another measure of the same phenomenon (if such exists) is used to compare the results from a new questionnaire. Predictive validity is the ability of the questionnaire to predict other related phenomena (Bowling, 1995). For example, using quality of life as an example, you could predict that people with poor quality of life may also be unhappy. The ultimate concept in validity is construct validity (Bowling, 1995; Eysenck, 1994), which encompasses the ability of the questionnaire to converge with other measures which may be related to the same phenomenon, such as age and sex, and discriminant validity whereby the questionnaire is able to discriminate from measures of other phenomena. Establishing the validity of a questionnaire is a tedious process but one which is essential if the utility of a questionnaire, leading to its subsequent use by others, is to be established.

STATISTICAL ANALYSIS

Some mention of statistics is unavoidable in a chapter which considers quantitative research methods. Statistical analysis is the means by which the quantitative researcher decides whether or not the results of a study represent a real phenomenon or whether they are spurious. However, for the purpose of this chapter, no expertise will be assumed and no effort to teach actual statistical methods will be made. The purpose behind the use of statistics and what some of the more common tests are used for will be conveyed.

In order to appreciate why statistical analysis is used alongside quantitative methods it is necessary to have a rudimentary understanding of the concept of probability. It is against the possibility of the results of a quantitative study occurring by chance that the quantitative researcher must guard. The probability of an event happening (p) is expressed as a number between zero and one i.e. $0<p<1$. In theory the probability of an event happening, no matter how unlikely, is never zero and, however likely, is never one (Walsh, 1990). Therefore, from the results of a quantitative study, the researcher wants to establish that the probability of what has been observed has only a very small probability of being observed. In other words, the observation has a high probability of being the result of the experiment or a relationship between two variables. Essentially, all statistical tests are designed to help the researcher come to a decision about the likelihood of an observation taking place by chance and an appropriate test should be selected (Robson, 1973).

Level of Significance

The level of significance is the probability of the outcome of a study being unlikely to have occurred by chance. Conventionally this is set at $p \leq 0.05$ which means that the probability of the outcome of a study occurring by chance is less that one in twenty or five per cent (Walsh, 1990). Failure to set an acceptably low level of statistical significance leads to Type I error which is acceptance of the outcome of an experiment or a relationship between variables as real when the observations are spurious (Walsh, 1990).

While computers have greatly aided the expedition of statistical tests, it is essential nevertheless to understand what the test is doing. All tests produce a number which can be located in a standard table of such values according to the number of subjects in the test and the desired level of significance in order to decide if the results of the study are statistically significant.

Statistical Tests

Three common statistical tests will be considered: the t-test, Pearson's correlation and the Chi-square test.

The t-test

The t-test compares the means of two groups in order to see if the difference between the means is statistically significant (Walsh, 1990). For example, referring to the example on caring which was used above, if a group of males and a group of females in nursing were asked to complete a questionnaire which measured caring then the difference between the mean scores for the groups could be tested for statistical significance using a t-test. The test would produce a value for t which would be located in a table of t values, as described above, to provide the statistical significance of the result.

Pearson's correlation

Pearson's correlation provides a measure of the strength of a relationship between two variables (Bryman and Cramer, 1997). It is also possible, as described above, to estimate the extent to which the relationship has occurred by chance. For example, if the level of knowledge of dementia and the length of time of working in care of the elderly were measured in a group of nurses then it could be hypothesised that there would be a relationship between these two variables. Using Pearson's correlation a value called r would be calculated and this indicates the strength of the relationship. Values of r greater than or equal to zero and less than or equal to one, i.e. $0 \leq r \leq 1$, with one indicating a perfect relationship and zero indicating no relationship. The value of r can be located on a table and the statistical significance of the relationship judged as described above. The word of caution given above regarding the interpretation of correlation will be reiterated: it is not possible to ascribe cause and effect unless the relationship between the two variables is clearly understood.

Chi-square

An example of where chi-square could be used would be to investigate a relationship between two nominal variables (Polit and Hungler, 1995). An example from nursing would be the possibility of a relationship between which part of the register nurses were on (e.g. general or psychiatric) and which hospital they worked in. A value of chi-square (χ^2) is calculated and located on a table of χ^2 values as described above in order to determine statistical significance.

CONCLUSION

Lord Kelvin is reputed to have said 'that which cannot be measured is not worth knowing' which is an extreme position. Nevertheless, measurement is a useful and essential component of nursing research provided that such aspects as level of measurement, reliability and validity, sample size and the application of appropriate tests for statistical significance are understood. Rather than agreeing wholeheartedly with Lord Kelvin, perhaps we should ensure that that which can be measured is measured, and measured well.

REFERENCES

Atkinson, F.I. (1996) Survey design and sampling, in: D.S.F. Cormack (ed), *The Research Process in Nursing*. London: Blackwell: 202–13.

Bowling, A. (1995) *Measuring Disease*. Buckingham: Open University Press.

Bryman, A. and Cramer, D. (1997*) Quantitative Data Analysis with SPSS for Windows: a Guide for Social Scientists*. London: Routledge.

Cohen, J. (1992) A power primer, *Psychological Bulletin*, 112: 155–9.

Eysenck, M.W. (1994) *Individual Differences: Normal and Abnormal*. Hove: Erlbaum.

Ferguson, E. and Cox, T. (1993) Exploratory factor analysis: a user's guide, *International Journal of Selection and Assessment*, 2: 84–95.

Jardine, J. (1964) *Physics is Fun*. London: Heinemann.

Kline, P. (1994) *An Easy Guide to Factor Analysis*. London: Routledge.

Lynn, M.R. (1986) Determination and quantification of content validity, *Nursing Research*, 35: 382–5.

Parahoo, K. (1997) *Nursing Research: Principles, Process and Issues*. London: Macmillan.

Polit, D.F. and Hungler, B.P. (1995) *Nursing Research* (5th edn). Philadelphia: Lippincott.

Robson, C. (1973) *Experiment, Design and Statistics in Psychology*. Harmondsworth: Penguin.

Seaton, M.A. Davidson, G.W. Schwartz, C.M., and Simpson, J. (1986*) Chambers 20th Century Thesaurus*. Edinburgh: Chambers.

Sheatsley, P.B. (1983) Questionnaire construction and item writing, in: P.H. Rossi, J.D Wright and A.B. Anderson (eds), *Handbook of Survey Research*. New York: Academic Press: 195–230.

Walsh, A. (1990) *Statistics for the Social Sciences: With Computer Applications*. Grand Rapids: Harper & Row.

Watson, R. and Kuhn, M. (1990) The influence of component parts on the performance of urinary sheath systems, *Journal of Advanced Nursing*, 15: 417–22.

Watson, R. and Lea, A. (1997) The caring dimensions inventory (CDI): content validity, reliability and scaling, *Journal of Advanced Nursing*, 25: 87–94.

5

The Research Critique

Therese Connell Meehan

The primary responsibility of the professional nurse is to give the best possible nursing care to individuals, families and groups – sick and well. To this end, nurses draw upon a range of ways of knowing what is most truthful and effective in nursing practice. Ways of knowing include faith, reason and science. Through integration of knowledge from these sources, each nurse as both a loving person and a thinking person engages in nursing practice – what Nightingale (1867 cited in Baly, 1991: 68) called 'one of the fine arts'.

Critiquing research is an integral part of knowing through science. The research critique is a process of critical reading and critical thinking through which the scientific merit of research studies and the validity of study findings are evaluated for the purpose of determining their value for practice and implications for further knowledge development. Evaluation is guided by logical thinking, knowledge of the research process and generally agreed upon standards, or criteria, for how to conduct valid or trustworthy research. The research critique serves as a crucial connection between the *thinking* and *doing* of nursing; between nursing science and the art of nursing practice. It facilitates continuous communication and exchange of questions, ideas, insights, judgements, answers and always more questions – all of which contribute, either directly or indirectly, to developing and improving nursing practice.

Thinking nurses cannot escape the fact that the nursing literature is replete with research reports related to nursing practice, education, management and public health policy. However, owing to the nature and restrictiveness of nursing education in the recent past and major changes which are currently occurring, there tends to be a variety of responses to the idea that, as a matter of course, all professional nurses are expected to read and evaluate research critically, use new knowledge appropriately and contribute to further knowledge development. In fact, ongoing critical evaluation of research reports and appropriate use of research findings are essential clinical skills, just as monitoring patients' needs for pain relief and providing patient education are essential clinical skills. The integration of all types of clinical skills plays an essential role in safe, appropriate and effective patient care. In this chapter questions related to the critical evaluation of research reports are discussed and the process of critiquing research is reviewed.

THE NATURE AND NECESSITY OF CRITICISM

The essence of the research critique is critical reading and critical thinking. However, for the beginning reader two questions may immediately come to mind: Is it right to be critical? and is criticism really necessary? Sometimes an initial response to the idea of being critical is to recoil from the thought of being negative and hurtful to others and, by association, the underlying fear of receiving such opprobrium oneself. But this is not at all what criticism means in the context of the research critique. Like many words, 'critical' has several different meanings. It is true that in everyday language 'critical' is often used in its meaning of 'adverse and unfavourable: fault-finding' (*The Oxford English Dictionary*, Vol. IV, 1989: 30) and so is associated with being severely judgmental or derogatory. However, in research and in all scholarly work 'critical' is always used in its meaning of 'involving or exercising careful judgement or observation; [being] exact, accurate, precise' (*The Oxford English Dictionary*, Vol. IV, 1989: 30). Here 'critical' refers to the art of estimating logically the quality and integrity of professional work and has two essential characteristics. One is questioning the meaning and credibility of ideas and actions and measuring them against standards or criteria with exacting precision and without prejudice. The other is that the critical approach is always impersonal and engaged in with sensitivity and kindness. Thus the research critique, as a process of critical reading and critical thinking, involves the reader in continually estimating the quality of research and exercising careful judgement with regard to its credibility and usefulness for professional practice. In this sense, being critical is the rightful responsibility of every professional nurse.

It may still be questioned, however, whether it is really necessary to be critical when reading nursing and other professional literature in general, and research literature in particular. It may be thought that surely with professional journals being so important, what is written in them must be carefully examined and verified before it is published – surely, busy practising nurses can rely on the professional literature to tell them what is best to do. But this is not necessarily the case. Underlying the idea of critical reading and critical thinking is the common-sense principle that you cannot believe everything that you are told – even by researchers.

While it is true that researchers are expected to evaluate critically their own work, and that research published in most professional journals has been critically evaluated by independent reviewers, the fact remains that not all published research is good research. Some research is credible and some research is less credible, and professional nurses who take direct responsibility for patient care must be able to distinguish between the two. So, it is necessary to be critical. Patient welfare and professional integrity depend upon it. Polgar and Thomas (1995: 343) underline the importance of this point when they propose that the reader's proper attitude to published research is 'hard-nosed scepticism'.

A PLAN FOR ACTION

In beginning a research critique, it is important to have a specific plan in mind which will ensure that the best use is made of available time and that the critique is as comprehensive as possible. There are several critiquing plans proposed in the literature, for example, Downs (1984), Scandlyn (1987), Topham and Silva (1988), Forchuck and Roberts (1993), Liehr and Houston (1993) and Hek (1996). LoBiondo-Wood et al. (1998) propose a particularly effective plan composed of four levels of reading and understanding: preliminary, comprehensive, analysis and synthesis. For each level, specific critical thinking and reading skills are stressed and each level successively leads to greater understanding of research reports and comprehensiveness of critiquing skill. Increase in critiquing skill at each level can be expected to occur over time with increased knowledge and experience.

To begin with, it is usually necessary to make a photocopy of the report to be critiqued and to have essential tools at hand: a sharp pencil for making notes on the copy of the report, a highlighter for emphasising important statements, a comprehensive research textbook and a dictionary.

Preliminary Level

The preliminary level entails an initial overview of the report. This enables the reader to gain quickly an impression of the report as a whole. The title and abstract of the report are read in detail and the body of the report is 'skimmed'. 'Skimming' (LoBiondo-Wood et al., 1998: 42) consists of reading the introduction – usually the first one or two paragraphs, the main heading of each section and one or two sentences at the beginning and end of each section, and the summary and conclusions presented in the last one or two paragraphs. The beginning reader will be able to identify whether or not the steps of the research process are evident in the abstract and section headings, and thus differentiate a research report from other types of publication such as a review, case report or discussion article. It will also be evident whether the research is quantitative or qualitative, or a combination of both. The more experienced reader will be able to determine the main study concepts or variables and the specific type of research design used.

As soon as reading begins, ideas, insights, and questions arise and flow swiftly through the mind. It is important to write them down straight away in the margins of the photocopy or on the back of the pages. Otherwise, some will vanish as quickly as they arose and be difficult to recall. LoBiondo-Wood et al. (1998) recommend highlighting the steps of the research process as they are identified, as well as key statements and any new words. New words, and also words and concepts the reader may be unsure of, can be looked up in a research textbook or dictionary.

Comprehensive Level

The comprehensive level requires greater depth of critical reading and understanding. The whole report is read with close attention from beginning to end. The beginning reader may find it necessary to do this more than once to gain a reasonably comprehensive understanding of the study. Again, it will be helpful to highlight and make notes about important concepts and statements. At this level it will become more clearly evident which words, concepts and key statements are fully under-stood and which are still unclear or not understood. It will be especially important for the beginning reader to take any extra time necessary to look these up in a textbook. In addition, LoBiondo-Wood et al. (1998) suggest that it may be necessary to look up other literature. For example, if a theoretical framework is used, further reading about it may be necessary to understand the study. Readers are also encouraged to discuss the study with others, especially lecturers and tutors, to obtain help with identifying and understanding the steps of the research process and how they are interrelated in the study as a whole. In order to consolidate comprehension of the study, readers are encouraged to summarise the report in their own words in a short paragraph.

Analysis Level

Once some degree of comprehension has been attained, readers are ready to begin the analysis level. Here emphasis is placed on identifying and examining each step of the research process in detail. It is at this level that critiquing guidelines are used to check systematically whether scientific standards have been met in each step. In applying critiquing criteria, LoBiondo-Wood et al. (1998) again recommend keeping a textbook close at hand to clarify, where necessary, understanding of the steps of the research process and critiquing criteria. Readers will also find it helpful to summarise each section of the report and their evaluation in their own words in one or two sentences.

Typically, beginning readers find that the first few times this level of understanding is attempted, it is difficult and frustrating. But this is a natural part of the process of learning any complex skill and it is very understandable and expected that beginning readers ask for help. In the end patience and perseverance will win for readers the necessary reading and critiquing skill and considerable, if initially unexpected, self-confidence.

Synthesis Level

Critical reading and thinking at the synthesis level bring the reader to focus again on understanding the research report as a whole, but in much greater depth than previously. Based on understanding gained through application of critiquing criteria to each step of the research process at the analysis level, the reader can now appraise the strengths (where all or most criteria are met) and limitations (where most criteria are not met) of the study as a whole. LoBiondo-Wood et al. (1998) liken this stage to looking at a completed jigsaw puzzle and considering whether all the pieces fit together or whether some pieces do not fit so well. The extent to which a study meets all the appropriate critiquing criteria indicates the extent to which the study findings are credible and, therefore, potentially useful. Readers are encouraged to briefly summarise the whole report and its overall strengths and limitations in their own words.

CRITIQUING GUIDELINES

The following guidelines and critiquing criteria, in the form of questions, are suggested for beginning readers. They follow the steps of the research process, which in reports are organised under section headings. Because quantitative and qualitative approaches to research arise from different philosophical perspectives, each reflects the steps of the research process in a different way. Thus, following initial critique of the study title, authors, abstract and funding, critique of quantitative and qualitative reports will be addressed separately.

Title, Abstract, Authors and Funding

A good title usually has about ten to fifteen words which indicate the specific focus of the research. The abstract should summarise the report in 100–200 words and include the main steps of the research process, some of which should be stated explicitly but some may be implied. The purpose, sample and its size, how data were collected and the major findings and conclusions should be stated explicitly. Research questions or hypotheses, the study design and type of data analyses may be stated but are often implied. Researchers' qualifications indicate the level of practice insight and research skill that can be expected in the report. Funding, as an indicator of quality, increases the probability that the study is credible.

- Is the title brief and clear?
- Does the title contain the major variables and population?
- Is the abstract brief and specific and provide a comprehensive summary of the study?
- What are the authors' academic and practice qualifications?
- Was the study funded?

Critiquing Quantitative Reports

Critiquing quantitative research is not always approached initially with great enthusiasm. Its emphasis on objectivity, numerical data, precision of measurement, probability theory, control and manipulation often do not resonate with nurses' mainly subjective perceptions of practice. However, critique of quantitative research is not as difficult as it first may appear and mastery of this skill is essential for nurses who seek to demonstrate clearly both the health and cost benefits of nursing care. Quantitative research plays a central role in determining public health policy and strategic planning for future needs. It is also the prevailing language of the Department of Health, the health care industry and other professional groups.

Problem, purpose and significance
The problem, the scope of the problem, and the need for the study (its significance) should be addressed clearly and objectively in the opening paragraphs. The purpose or reason why the study was conducted should be stated explicitly either at the end of the introduction or the end of the literature review.

- Is the problem stated clearly, concisely and objectively in the opening paragraphs?
- Are the study variables and population included in the problem statement?
- If the problem includes more than one variable, is it clear how they relate to one another?
- Is the problem significant for nursing practice and health care?
- Is the purpose of the study clearly identified?
- Are the problem and purpose congruent with one another?

Literature review

It should be clear that the study is <u>being conducted in relation to what</u> is already known and <u>not yet known about the problem</u> and that it <u>builds</u> <u>on findings of previous studies</u>. Generally, quoted material and <u>subjective</u> <u>experiences</u> should not be included, and <u>personal opinion never</u> <u>included</u>. The review should consist of a logically organised and critical examination of relevant previous studies and conclude with a summary of what is known and not yet known about the study problem. This, in turn, <u>should lead</u> to the <u>identification of a gap</u> in knowledge about the problem that the current study is designed to fill and the consequent need for the study.

- Is the literature review <u>comprehensive</u>?
- Is the review <u>concise</u> and <u>logically presented</u>?
- Are the study variables defined specifically?
- Are <u>mainly primary sources cited</u>?
- Are all the sources <u>relevant</u> to the study problem and variables?
- Are current and older sources included appropriately?
- Are <u>conflicting results from previous studies</u> indicated?
- Is a critical evaluation of previous studies presented?
- <u>Is the literature review summarised</u>?
- Is the gap in the literature to be filled by the current study identified?

Theoretical framework

If a theoretical framework is included, it should contribute significantly to understanding of the problem and how the study variables relate to or affect one another. It should guide all the steps of the research process, particularly the definition and measurement of variables. A theoretical framework usually provides a basis for stating hypotheses rather than asking research questions.

- Is a <u>theoretical framework</u> used and is it clearly identified?
- Is the theoretical framework from nursing or another discipline?
- Does the theoretical framework describe the problem adequately and explain relationships among the variables?
- Does the theoretical framework guide the definition and measure-ment of the study variables?
- Does the theoretical framework guide the statement of hypotheses?

Research questions and hypotheses

The study problem and purpose, having been examined through the review of literature and theoretical framework if one is used, should lead logically to the research questions or hypotheses. Research questions are appropriate in exploratory descriptive studies, or in comparative and correlational studies where only a few previous studies related to the problem are reported and not much is yet known about it in scientific terms. Hypotheses are appropriate in studies which explain or predict relationships or effects among variables and especially when a theoretical framework consistent with previous research findings is used.

- Does the report contain research questions or hypotheses? –No clear
- Do the research questions or hypotheses follow clearly from the study problem?
- Are the research questions or hypotheses stated explicitly or implied?
- Are the research questions or hypotheses clear and concise?
- Do the research questions or hypotheses contain the study variables and population?
- Are the research questions or hypotheses appropriate for the study?
- What are the independent and dependent variables in each research question or hypothesis?
- For hypotheses, does each contain only one predicted result so that it is either supported or not supported in the statistical analysis?
- For hypotheses, are they scientifically testable?

Design and methods

Each type of research question or hypothesis leads logically to a specific type of research design. Each type of design, in turn, leads to specific methods of data collection and analysis. The main purpose of a research design is to control as much as is practically possible for the influence of extraneous variables, that is, threats to internal and external study validity which could bring about false results.

- Is the design stated explicitly or implied?
- Is the design experimental or non-experimental?
- Is the design appropriate for answering the research questions or testing the hypotheses?
- If intervention and control groups are used, are the steps of the intervention and control procedures defined in detail?
- Does the study design allow researchers to claim cause and effect relationships among the study variables?
- Does the design include as much control as possible for the influence of extraneous variables and other threats to internal and external study validity?
- Are the limitations of the design identified?

Methods: sample and setting

Every effort should have been made, within the restrictions imposed by the type of problem and design and the exigencies of the study setting, to ensure that the sample is not biased and represents the population as closely as possible. A general description of the institution or community where the study was conducted should be given so readers can evaluate whether the study setting seems appropriate and how similar or different it is to their own practice settings.

- Is the population accessible to the researchers described?
- What inclusion or exclusion criteria were used to select a homogeneous sample?
- Was sample selection non-random or random?
- Were all members of the population who met the criteria for inclusion invited to participate in the study or included in the randomisation process?
- Is the sampling method consistent with the study design?
- Is the sample size stated?
- Is a rationale given for sample size and is the size adequate?
- If subjects were assigned to groups, was assignment random or non-random?
- Were any subjects lost from the sample during data collection and the reasons for their loss reported?
- Are the characteristics of the sample described in some detail?
- Is enough information provided for readers to judge if the sample is biased? *Cross sectional may be biased*
- How well does the sample represent the population?
- Is the study setting described?

Methods: protection of human subjects

Every research report must include confirmation that *subjects*, or their *legal guardians*, gave their informed, usually written, consent to participate and were ensured of the anonymity or confidentiality of the data they provided. If subjects were from a vulnerable population such as hospitalised patients, the elderly, children, pregnant women, the unborn, or the emotionally, mentally or physically disabled, additional information should be given about how their basic human rights were protected.

- Is it stated that subjects or their legal guardians gave informed, usually written, consent to participate?
- Was anonymity or confidentiality of data assured?
- If vulnerable subjects were used, was additional assurance given that their basic human rights were protected?
- Is there any indication that subjects, or their legal guardians, did not understand the nature of the study or were coerced to participate in the study?

Methods: measurement

In quantitative research, experiences and events in the form of variables are converted into numerical data so that they can be measured objectively. This process of data collection and measurement must be conducted and reported with exacting logic and precision in order to ensure that the measurement methods used were accurately and consistently measuring what they were supposed to measure. If validity and reliability of measurement methods are not reasonably assured the study results have little meaning.

• What type of data collection and measurement methods were used?
• Were the data collection and measurement methods clearly described?
• If an instrument or measurement method was designed specifically for the study, is its development fully described and its validity and reliability established?
• Were the data collection and measurement methods appropriate for use in the study?
• Was evidence of at least two types of validity given for each measurement method?
• Was evidence of at least two types of reliability given for each measurement method?
• What level of measurement was used for each variable?
• Was the highest appropriate level of measurement used for each variable?

Methods: procedures for data collection

Consistency of data collection procedures is essential to control for threats to study validity owing to variations in data collection procedures. Data should be collected from all subjects in the same manner. If more than one person collected data, assurance should be given that they were collecting the data in the same way. This is called inter-rater reliability. Researchers conducting clinical studies should not themselves provide study treatments or collect data because of their potential to personally influence subjects' responses. However, for logistic reasons they often do and readers need to judge the extent to which this biased the study results.

• Is who collected the data and how, where and when it was collected clearly described?
• Were data collected in the same manner and place and during the same type of time period for all subjects?
• If more than one person collected the data, was inter-rater reliability demonstrated?
• If researchers administered study interventions or collected their data, did they explain how they minimised resulting bias?

Data analysis and results

In quantitative research, data analysis and results inevitably mean statistics and these can range from simple to very complex. This section of the report should be brief and to the point with any discussion of the results left to the discussion section. It may be difficult for beginning readers to critique statistical analyses and results, especially if they have not taken a statistics course. Most readers will wish to keep a textbook close at hand and be ready to make notes about needs for additional assistance.

- What descriptive statistics are reported?
- Are the descriptive statistics appropriate for levels of measurement?
- Are inferential statistics reported?
- Are the inferential statistics appropriate for levels of measurement of variables, sample size, and the type of research questions or hypotheses?
- Is the level of significance stated and, if so, what is it?
- Are the main results clearly and concisely presented for each research question or hypothesis?
- If tables or figures are used, are they presented clearly, labelled accurately and informative?
- If tables or figures are used, do they complement the text and not repeat it?

Discussion

The discussion should be objective and based on a logical and discerning interpretation of the results. Results should be interpreted in light of the study limitations and compared and contrasted with results of previous studies of the problem, particularly those reported in the literature review. It should not include personal opinion. Results that are expected should be interpreted conservatively and with caution and any possible alternative explanations presented. If expected results are not obtained, discussion of possible reasons this occurred should be presented. Discussion should also include the meaning and appropriate use of the results for nursing and health care as well as their implications for further research. For studies concerned with clinical practice, the statistical and clinical significance of the results should be compared. Finally, conclusions should be stated indicating the final meaning and worth of the results.

- Is the discussion presented in an objective and logical manner?
- Is each research question or hypothesis addressed?
- Are the limitations of the study identified?
- Are the results discussed in light of the limitations of the study?
- Are the results compared and contrasted with results of previous studies cited in the literature review?
- If a theoretical framework was used, how are the results related to it?

- Are implications for practice, theory development, education, management or health policy discussed as appropriate?
- Are recommendations made for further research?
- What conclusions are made?
- Are the conclusions supported by the results or do they extend beyond what the results actually indicate?

Critiquing Qualitative Reports

Critiquing qualitative research is usually appealing because it concerns subjective experiences and their meaning and is reported in narrative form. Most nurses have some personal resonance with this kind of data and feel it is more authentic. However in critiquing, care must be taken not to be swayed by subjective appeal. Hinds et al. (1990: 403) follow Miles and Huberman (1984) in warning that 'qualitative research findings can be evocative, illuminating, masterful and wrong'. It must be kept in mind that although qualitative research is primarily subjective, objectivity in its evaluation is essential.

Phenomenon of interest, purpose and significance
The phenomenon of interest – what is being studied – should be made clear in the opening paragraphs. Frequently, this is achieved through the use of quoted statements which illustrate the nature of the human experience or social process of interest from the perspective of individuals experiencing it. It should also be clear that greater understanding of the phenomenon and its meaning are important for improving the quality of nursing and health care. The purpose, or reason why the study was conducted, should be stated explicitly at the end of the introduction. The purpose and how it is conceptualised determine the type of qualitative approach chosen and how the steps of the research process are implemented.

- Is the phenomenon of interest stated clearly and concisely in the opening paragraphs?
- Is the phenomenon of interest significant for nursing and health care?
- Is the purpose of the study clearly identified?
- Is it clear why a qualitative approach is being used to examine the phenomenon?

Literature review
Occasionally, no literature review will be presented prior to the conduct of a qualitative study. However, a brief review is usually included to help focus the study, more fully define the phenomenon of interest and

outline what is not yet known about it. Usually, previous research and other literature are examined more fully in the discussion section.

- Is a literature review included prior to the conduct of the study?
- Does the literature review help focus the study?
- Does the literature review enhance understanding of the phenomenon of interest?
- Are all the sources relevant to the phenomenon of interest?
- Is a critical evaluation of the literature presented?
- Is a summary of the literature presented?
- Is the gap in the literature to be filled by the current study identified?

Research question
Qualitative research is always guided by a research question, never an hypothesis. The question should be consistent with the phenomenon of interest and purpose and lead logically to the particular type of research approach that is used. It should be noted that the emergent, fluid nature of qualitative research will sometimes lead to a change in the study's phenomenon of interest and purpose and reformulation of the research question. This is acceptable as long as the process is explained and the restated phenomenon of interest, purpose and research question are consistent with one another.

- Does the research question encompass the phenomenon of interest?
- Is the research question consistent with the phenomenon of interest and study purpose?

Methods: research approach
There are at least 20 different approaches to qualitative research which are differentiated according to different philosophical perspectives or sets of philosophical assumptions. The particular approach being used in a study – for example, ethnographic, grounded theory, hermeneutic or phenomenological – should be stated explicitly and the philosophical assumptions underlying the approach clearly identified. Each approach leads logically to specific methods of data collection.

- Is the specific qualitative approach used for the study clearly identified?
- Are the philosophical assumptions underlying the approach described and explained?
- Is the research approach consistent with the phenomenon of interest and the purpose?
- Are data collection methods which are consistent with the approach identified and followed?
- Are the data collection methods consistent with the philosophical assumptions underlying the approach?

Methods: sample and setting
Purposive sampling is usually most appropriate for two reasons: researchers should deliberately choose participants who they are sure have experienced, or are centrally involved in, the phenomenon of interest, and participants should be the persons available who are most able to articulate or exemplify the phenomenon of interest. Other sampling methods are used in special circumstances. A rationale for the sample size and its adequacy should be given; these are usually determined by data saturation. The study setting is of particular importance in qualitative research because it is often the natural environment of the study participants and where they experience the phenomenon of interest. Where researchers were present in the setting, they should give assurance that it was altered as little as possible by their presence and conduct of the study. Where participants were interviewed about experiences that occurred at a prior time, the interview setting should be described and should usually be similar for all participants.

- Is the population accessible to the researcher described?
- What sampling method was used and was it appropriate for the specific research approach?
- Were the participants appropriate for answering the research question?
- How was the sample size determined?
- Was the sample size adequate?
- Are the characteristics of the sample described in some detail?
- Is the study setting, or interview setting, described?

Methods: protection of research participants
There are very few circumstances where informed consent and assurance of confidentiality are not required for *all participants* or their *legal guardians*, including complex field settings and the use of participant observation techniques. If subjects were from a vulnerable population such as hospitalised patients, the elderly, children, pregnant women, the unborn, or the emotionally, mentally or physically disabled, additional information should be given about how their basic human rights were protected. If any changes are made in the research process, participants should be informed and their further consent obtained.

- Is it stated that all participants or their legal guardians gave their informed, usually written, consent to participate?
- Were all participants assured of confidentiality?
- If vulnerable subjects were used, was additional assurance given that their basic human rights were protected?
- If the data collection process was altered or extended, was additional consent obtained?

- Is there any indication that participants, or their legal guardians, did not understand the nature of the study or were coerced to participate in the study?

Methods: role of the researcher

In qualitative approaches researchers are subjectively involved in every step of the data collection and analysis. In particular, through interviews or observations and their analyses of recorded data, they are subjectively involved in interpreting all information given by respondents. Because these circumstances allow so much potential for researchers to influence the data personally, it is important that their data collection activities are made as clear as possible. During the research process, researchers are required to become as consciously aware as possible of their own thoughts, attitudes and personal beliefs about the study topic. A brief summary of these should be included in the report and researchers are usually expected to confirm that they 'bracketed' them, thereby consciously excluding them as much as possible from the process of data collection and analysis. For some qualitative research approaches where this concept is not recognised as being important, readers must consider carefully the extent to which the study results may represent the perceptions of the researcher rather than those of the participants, and the implications of this situation.

- Has the researcher made clear his or her thoughts, perceptions and feelings concerning the phenomenon of interest?
- Was assurance given that these were bracketed during data collection and analysis?

Methods: data collection and analysis

Both the process and specific methods of data collection and analysis should be described in detail. Each type of research approach leads to the use of particular data collection methods or combinations of methods. Similarly, each type of research approach specifies particular methods of analysis. Readers should check carefully that these were followed. Usually, data collection and data analysis proceed simultaneously. It should be clear how the researchers condensed the data into the themes, categories and summary statements used to describe the essential features of the experience or social process of interest.

- Is the data collection process fully described?
- What data collection methods were used?
- Are the data collection methods clearly described?
- Is the data recording process described?
- Are the data collection methods consistent with the purpose of the study and the specific research approach being used?

- Was the data collection process comprehensive?
- Are the strategies used to analyse the data described?
- Are the data collection process and strategies used to analyse data consistent with the purpose of the study?
- Was data saturation reached?

Results

Qualitative research results are, of course, narrative. They should be presented in themes or categories or both, as specified by the research approach. The verity of each theme or category should be substantiated by illustrative quotes from the participants. These data should lead to a final statement which fully answers the research question. Summary results may be presented as a written description of an experience or presented as a diagram of a conceptual schema or theory of a social process.

- Are the results described systematically?
- Are the derived themes or categories clearly presented?
- Is the verity of the derived themes or categories substantiated?
- Are the relationships between the themes or categories clear?
- Did the data lead to the type of results that are consistent with the specific research approach?
- Do the results communicate the phenomenon of interest and its meaning as it is experienced by the participants vividly and profoundly?
- Has the research question been fully answered?

Methods: data trustworthiness

The credibility of qualitative research, referred to as trustworthiness, is judged according to the carefulness and precision with which data are analysed and the closeness of the final results to both the participants' and others' experience of the phenomenon. Trustworthiness can be judged according to three criteria: credibility, dependability (auditability) and transferability (fittingness).

- Are the procedures used to establish the credibility of the data described?
- Is the creditability of the data adequate?
- Are the procedures used to establish the dependability of the data described?
- Is the dependability of the data adequate?
- Is the transferability of the data demonstrated?

Discussion

Although the conduct of qualitative research is a subjective process, discussion of the results should be objective and carefully reasoned. A review of literature related to the phenomenon of interest should be incorporated into the discussion, especially if it has not been presented earlier, and the study results should be compared and contrasted with what was previously known about the study problem. It is important that study limitations, although they may have been unavoidable, are identified and their implications for the results discussed. The final meaning and worth of the results should be summarised with caution, and implications for further research and theory development stated. Readers should keep in mind that while results of qualitative studies cannot be generalised to other similar populations, they can be extremely valuable in enhancing understanding of the human experiences and social processes inherent in nursing practice situations.

- Is the discussion presented in an objective manner?
- Is a comprehensive literature review included?
- Are the limitations of the study identified and the results discussed in light of the limitations?
- Are the results compared and contrasted with the findings of previous studies and other literature?
- Are implications for practice and theory development discussed?
- Are recommendations made for further research?
- What conclusions are made?
- Are the conclusions supported by the results or do they extend beyond what the results actually indicate?

CONCLUSION

Professional nurses draw upon different types of knowledge to guide their practice, including knowledge generated through scientific inquiry. All are expected to critique research reports and determine their credibility and usefulness for professional practice. Beginning readers are entreated not to give in to feeling overwhelmed by the considerable amount of detailed work which the research critique appears to call for. Like any clinical skill, it is simply a matter of practice.

As an analogy, readers might recall their experience as student nurses of being on the wards for the first time. The new language and skills required to care for patients sometimes led to feelings of helplessness and never being able to cope. But in no time at all the new language and skills were second nature. So it is with critiquing research reports for the first time. Beginning experiences may be difficult but with patience and perseverance critiquing research also becomes second nature. The habit of critical reading and critical thinking sharpens the mind. The nurse as a loving person with a sharp mind is immeasurably equipped to give the best possible nursing care in all circumstances.

REFERENCES

Downs, F. (1984) Elements of a research critique, in: F. Downs (ed.), *Nursing Research: Addresses, Essays, Lectures*. Philadelphia: F.A. Davis.

Edgerton, S. (1998) Guide to critique of philosophical research, in: C. Hoskins (ed.), *Developing Research in Nursing and Health*. New York: Springer: 119.

Forchuck, C. and Roberts, J. (1993) How to critique qualitative research articles, *Canadian Journal of Nursing Research*, 25 (4): 47–56.

Hek, G. (1996) Guidelines on conducting a critical research evaluation, *Nursing Standard*, 11 (6): 40–3.

Hinds, P., Scandrett-Hibden, S., and McAulay, L. (1990) Further assessment of a method to estimate reliability and validity of qualitative research finding, *Journal of Advanced Nursing*, 13: 430–5.

Liehr, P. and Houston, S. (1993) Critiquing and using nursing research: guidelines for the critical care nurse, *American Journal of Critical Care*, 2 (5): 407–12.

LoBiondo-Wood, G., Haber, J., and Krainovich-Miller, B. (1998) Overview of the research process, in: G. LoBiondo-Wood and J. Haber (eds), *Nursing Research: Methods, Critical Appraisal and Utilization*, 4th edn. St Louis: Mosby.

Miles, M. & Huberman, A. (1984) *Qualitative Data Analysis: A Sourcebook of New Methods*. Beverley Hills CA: Sage.

Nightingale, F. (1867) To the editor, *Macmillan's Magazine*, April, cited in Baly, M. (ed.) (1991) *As Miss Nightingale Said . . .* London: Scutari.

Polgar, S and Thomas, S. (1995) *Introduction to Research in the Health Sciences*. Melbourne: Churchill Livingstone.

Scandlyn, J. (1987) How to read a research article, *Orthopaedic Nursing*, 6 (5): 21–7.

The Oxford English Dictionary, Vol. IV, 2nd edn (1989) Oxford: Clarendon.

Topham, D. and DeSilva, P. (1988) Evaluating congruency between steps in the research process: A critique guide for use in clinical nursing practice, *Clinical Nurse Specialist*, 2 (2): 97–102.

6
Research Utilisation
Gerard M. Fealy

INTRODUCTION

Research utilisation is that interaction between research knowledge and the sphere of practice, in which there is transfer of research-based knowledge into practice. This chapter explores research utilisation both as a concept and as a practical endeavour. It discusses the nature of research utilisation and it explores the factors that influence the utilisation of research. The chapter recounts the nursing experience with research utilisation and discusses the roles and responsibilities of key personnel in the process of implementing the findings of research in clinical nursing practice. Additionally, the chapter identifies a number of important research utilisation models that have been advanced in the light of experiences with research utilisation. Action research is proposed as an alternative research utilisation model.

Research Utilisation: A Professional Imperative

The utilisation of research findings in clinical practice is seen as being important in improving patient outcomes, enhancing the environment of professional practice and containing health care costs (Titler et al., 1994). Research-based practice is justified on grounds of professionalism, accountability, quality of care and cost-effectiveness (Bircumshaw, 1990). Research utilisation equates with evidence-based practice (Meehan, 1998), which refers to that practice that is based upon best available evidence of its effectiveness in attaining the best possible client outcomes. Evidence-based practice aims at promoting more clinically effective care (Kitson, 1997). Clinical effectiveness, through evidence-based practice, is a means of assuring quality of care for clients. Research utilisation is thus integrally linked to quality assurance (Meehan, 1997).

Research is seen as being '. . . an integral part of all aspects of nursing and midwifery' (Government of Ireland, 1998: 113), and research-based practice is viewed as being fundamental to the future of nursing as an autonomous practice-based discipline (Hancock, 1993). The International Council of Nurses (ICN) has pointed to the impact of nursing research on health care worldwide, including the identification of effective models of health care, significant benefits from patient teaching, improved quality of nursing care, reduced mortality and cost effectiveness (Mead, 1996). Research utilisation is therefore of immense concern to individual practitioners and to the nursing profession more generally.

DEFINING RESEARCH UTILISATION

Research utilisation has been referred to as the vehicle that carries scientific knowledge to the client (Goode et al., 1991). The process involves the identification of a practice problem, the identification of research knowledge related to the problem, the transfer of that knowledge into clinical decisions and actions and the evaluation of the effects of those decisions and actions.

Polit and Hungler (1995) point to a distinction between conceptual research utilisation and instrumental research utilisation. Conceptual utilisation refers to the way that practitioners are influenced in their thinking by their knowledge of research, but do not put this knowledge to any specific use. Conceptual research utilisation is important in the sense that it can extend the way that nurses think about what they do (Closs and Cheater, 1994), and it can lead nurses to cumulative understanding of different aspects of nursing practice (Meehan, 1997). Instrumental utilisation refers to that practice that is directly influenced by specific research knowledge. Instrumental utilisation means that certain actions are taken in the light of research knowledge and is the ideal type, since it ultimately leads to research-based practice (Meehan, 1997). Conceptual utilisation represents use of knowledge by the individual, whilst instrumental utilisation may be dependent upon factors outside of the individual's control, including factors in the work organisation (Lacey, 1994).

The Process of Research Utilisation

The process of research utilisation has been variously defined as an individual process (Stetler et al., 1995), as a decision-making process (Hunt, 1996), and as a group and an organisational process (Horsley et al., 1983). Practising nurses may arrive at research-based practice either through the identification of a clinical problem or through knowledge of the relevant research from the literature (Polit and Hungler, 1995). It is important to note that the process of research utilisation is not about basing clinical practice on the evidence of a single study (Goode et al.,

1991). Rather, it involves the identification of evidence from multiple research studies in a variety of sites and settings (Goode et al., 1991), and the synthesis of these studies in a single conceptual area (Horsley et al., 1983).

Horsley et al. (1983) describe the research utilisation process in terms of a planned organisational change, involving the identification of a clinical problem, the identification and assessment of multiple research studies related to the problem and the adaptation, design and clinical trial of practice innovations based on the research evidence. The process also includes decision making regarding the adoption, alteration or rejection of the innovation, extending the new or altered practice beyond the clinical trial site and maintaining the innovation over time. Hunt (1996) portrays research utilisation as a decision-making process, in which key decisions need to be taken at various stages in the process. A key decision in the early stage of research utilisation is whether or not to take action, having identified the practice problem or the relevant research knowledge. Decisions are also required in the selection of the appropriate client group and clinical setting in which to introduce change in response to the research evidence. When the practice innovation has been implemented and evaluated, further decisions are required with regard to the need to take further action.

MacGuire (1990) views the process of research utilisation as an aspect of the management of change and points to the fact that change is a complex and little understood process, with organisational change being particularly complex. This complexity is a function of the fact that individuals may have divergent goals and there may be resistance to change, since it requires that individuals alter their patterns of practice (MacGuire, 1990). The complexity of the task of achieving change should not be underestimated, since it introduces risks, it requires time and expenditure, it alters relationships and it possibly alters the status of individuals (Humphris, 1997).

RESEARCH UTILISATION: THE NURSING EXPERIENCE

Despite the proliferation of research, there is evidence that there is only sporadic use of research in clinical practice (Parahoo, 1997). In the 1980s a number of researchers reported poor or absent utilisation of research by nurses (Griffith, 1987; Murray, 1988; Deacon, 1986). Evidence from the 1990s suggests that research utilisation in clinical practice continued to be poor (Parahoo, 1998; Camiah, 1997; Webb and Mackenzie, 1993). Webb and Mackenzie (1993) studied research utilisation in relation to pre-operative fasting, pain assessment and pre-operative skin preparation, and found that the majority of nurses were not using research findings in practice, despite the wealth of research evidence available in relation to the three aspects of practice that were considered. Camiah (1997) reported the results of a case study on research utilisation in nursing practice, and found that many aspects of clinical nursing care were perceived by nurses as being '. . . largely affected by traditional beliefs and routine tasks' (Camiah, 1997: 1196). Aspects of nursing care, such as pre-operative fasting, pre-operative shaving, routine drug administration, pressure area care and the recording of vital signs were reported as being non-research based practice. On the basis of evidence from this study, Camiah concluded that '. . . routine and task-oriented nursing practice is still largely practised and valued despite a wide range of relevant research findings' (1997: 1196).

Parahoo (1998) reported the results of a large-scale survey on research utilisation among nurses in Northern Ireland. From a sample of 1,368 nurses, drawn from a wide variety of clinical settings, Parahoo (1998) reported that only about one third of the respondents reported utilising research either 'frequently' or 'all the time'. Furthermore, considerably less than half the sample reported having implemented new research findings in the two years prior to the survey. These self-reported practices were evident, despite very positive attitudes to research among the sample. Parahoo (1998: 290) concluded that research utilisation '. . . has yet to become a reality on a significant scale'. In a case study on the practice of continence promotion, Kevelighan (1994) explored research knowledge attainment and utilisation among a sample of eight qualified nurses in the Irish Republic. Kevelighan (1994) found that nurses who had participated in a continence promotion course had difficulty assimilating knowledge for continence promotion into both their thinking and their practice. Self-reported practices indicated that knowledge utilisation was moderated by the methods of care delivery and it appears that attempts to change practice were perceived as being a great disruption to the routine of care delivery.

While there is much evidence that many nurses fail to utilise research in practice, there is some counter-evidence pointing to research utilisation amongst nurses. Camiah (1997) found that nurses were using research in practice related to pain management, catheterisation and the admission of patients to hospital, and concluded that nurses were beginning to value the place of research in practice. Evidence from the self-reported practices of nurses in a pilot study conducted by Lacey (1994) indicated that nurses were routinely using research related to wound care protocols and pressure area care. In a survey of nearly three hundred nurses, Brett (1987) found that the majority were aware of practice innovations based on research, were persuaded by these innovations and used these innovations at least sometimes.

Notwithstanding these self-reported practices, evidence continues to emerge that there is a gap between knowledge generation and knowledge utilisation in nursing. If it is the case that there is widespread under-utilisation of research, then what are the factors that contribute to this situation? The following section will attempt to address this question.

FACTORS INFLUENCING RESEARCH UTILISATION

Much has been written about the factors that influence the utilisation of research in practice and a considerable amount of research has been conducted in order to explore and explain these factors. While the individual practitioner is ultimately responsible for effecting research utilisation in practice, the factors that influence the process of research utilisation are complex, with many residing outside the immediate control and professional jurisdiction of the individual practitioner.

Factors Related to the Communication and Dissemination of Research

Research utilisation requires dissemination, a process through which research findings are communicated to a wider audience. Early studies on research utilisation in nursing indicate that nurses did not have access to research literature (Myco, 1980; Miller and Messenger, 1978), and that nurses tended to be poor readers of professional literature (Myco, 1980). In the 1990s it seems that there is an information overload for nurses (Carter, 1996), with the sheer volume of research evidence available making finding and appraising a difficult task for the most committed practitioner (Mead, 1996).

These communication and availability problems may be compounded by the fact that research reports can employ a perspective with which many practitioners are unfamiliar (Alderton, 1983). Researchers may be producing research which meets the requirements of academic rigour, but which may not be addressing the immediate needs of practitioners. Many practitioners can perceive research as being esoteric and irrelevant to their everyday experiences and concerns (Kitson et al., 1996; Webb and MacKenzie, 1993). Furthermore, many nurses can find the language of research difficult to comprehend and many feel incapable of evaluating the quality of research (Dunn et al., 1998). Unfamiliar terminology can adversely affect understanding, and many nurses may not possess the skills needed to make decisions about which research issues are of relevance to their practice. As Parahoo (1997: 377) observed: 'The best studies are of little value if they are incomprehensible to those who could benefit most from them – the practitioners'.

Organisational Factors

It has been acknowledged that research utilisation is an organisational, rather than an individual process (Kitson et al., 1996). Research utilisation also has an interdisciplinary dimension (Rodgers, 1994). In attempting to implement research-based practices, nurses may encounter organisational barriers, such as resistance from other professional groups. Many nurses may perceive a lack of autonomy or may in fact lack autonomy, when it comes to altering clinical protocols, and may encounter opposition or non-cooperation from medical staff and nursing colleagues (Dunn et al., 1998; Rodgers, 1994; Lacey, 1994). This perceived lack of autonomy may be compounded by a perceived lack of cooperation from medical and administrative staff, which can frustrate clinicians' efforts at practice innovation (Rodgers, 1994).

The organisational climate would also appear to be an important factor in research utilisation. Two features of the organisational climate are important in relation to research utilisation in nursing. The first is concerned with managerial values and priorities, such as the relative emphasis placed on fiscal policies and professional practice, and the impact of these on service delivery. In this regard, Kenrick and Luker (1996) have instanced the growth of a managerial ethos within the National Health Service in the United Kingdom, which can undermine professional values. The second feature of organisational climate is the actual practice milieu within which nurses work. The everyday pressures of clinical practice, related to levels of client dependencies and levels of human and material resources, can reduce the clinician's enthusiasm for practice innovation and many nurses complain of a lack of time to implement research findings (Dunn et al., 1998).

Educational Factors

The demands of research utilisation are such that practitioners require a well-developed repertoire of intellectual and practical capacities, including skills related to research critiquing, clinical decision making and practice innovation and change. These intellectual capacities for research utilisation need to be complemented by a repertoire of clinical skills, as well as positive attitudes and professional values. Nurse education may be partially responsible for the non-utilisation of research in practice, in its failure to develop in the learner the requisite capacities for research utilisation. This failure may be related to the fact that research has been largely taught as a separate subject in the curriculum, with the emphasis on 'how to do it' (Parahoo, 1997). While learning about the research process is necessary for developing critical reading abilities, it does not in and of itself develop the sort of research-mindedness needed for research utilisation (Hunt, 1987). The failure of educators to integrate research findings into all areas of theoretical and clinical teaching content is seen as being an important reason why nurses are not sufficiently research minded and therefore not fervent users of research.

Individual Factors

While individual practitioners may possess the wherewithal to analyse research critically in terms of its appropriateness and validity, they may not be sufficiently motivated to base their practice on research (McKenna, 1995). Research utilisation assumes that nurses make free choices in the delivery of care (Rodgers, 1994). Choices are based upon disposition, beliefs and attitudes. The attitudes of nurse practitioners are especially important in determining whether research utilisation will happen. Champion and Leach (1989) found that negative attitudes were strongly related to research utilisation, while Hefferin et al. (1982) found that when nurses viewed research as being irrelevant to their practice, they were not motivated to spend time and effort on application. It also appears that nurses do not value research conducted by their own peers as much as research conducted by other health care professionals (Hicks, 1997).

Along with attitudes, role-concept appears to be an important factor in research utilisation. Lacey (1994) reported that nurses' self-perceived role was important to the attainment of research utilisation. Nurses who felt that they had a degree of autonomy in their clinical practice were more confident of their ability to change their practice, and being unable to challenge medical colleagues and organisational administrators represented the greatest deterrent to research utilisation. It appears that, at the level of the individual, research utilisation involves issues of autonomy and empowerment (Rodgers, 1994).

Research utilisation is a complex intellectual process involving knowledge assimilation and knowledge utilisation. This complexity may in and of itself militate against successful research utilisation. In this regard, Kevelighan (1994: 130) notes that '. . . the assimilation of new knowledge, even on topics directly related to practice, may be a difficult process for nurses'.

ROLES AND RESPONSIBILITIES IN RESEARCH UTILISATION

Research utilisation is a highly complex interdisciplinary undertaking that involves the participation of numerous individuals and resources (Closs and Cheater, 1994). In the light of the factors that act to impede research utilisation, it is evident that four key groups have roles and responsibilities in the process of research utilisation. These key groups are researchers, nurse managers, nurse educators and nurse practitioners.

The Role of the Researcher

While research reports should be presented in ways that uphold high academic and professional standards, researchers need to consider their use of language carefully when communicating their research findings. Research reports that are overloaded with research jargon will be confusing for the practising nurse who is uninitiated into the language of research (McKenna, 1995). The success of research utilisation is also determined by the extent to which researchers meet the needs of clinical staff (Kitson et al., 1996). Researchers need to show an understanding of the practitioners' everyday problems and concerns, through the identification of research questions that have their genesis in everyday practice. This can be achieved through greater researcher-practitioner collaboration, involving negotiation with clinical staff, in relation to the identification of clinical issues, and the setting of objectives and time frames for practice development (Kitson et al., 1996). The content of nursing research needs to include more studies that evaluate the outcomes of nursing interventions, including studies that demonstrate cost-effectiveness and quality of care (McKenna, 1995). Furthermore, researchers need to spell out the meanings of their results as well as the limitations of their application (Edwards-Beckett, 1990). In reporting and disseminating their findings, researchers need to include clear discussions about the relevance and potential usefulness of research (McKenna, 1995) and they need to present realistic proposals and plans for change (Closs and Cheater, 1994).

The Role of the Nurse Manager

Nurse managers can do much to bring about the organisational and practice changes that are required for research utilisation. In facilitating change, managers need to permit nurses to question their practice and to take chances with new research-based knowledge (McKenna, 1995). Nurse managers can promote research utilisation by fostering a climate of intellectual curiosity amongst nurses, by offering both moral and material support, and by rewarding efforts at research utilisation (Polit and Hungler, 1995). Furthermore, the time required for practice innovation must be promoted as legitimate use of staff time and the process of research application should be incorporated into the organisation's culture rather than being superimposed upon it (McKenna, 1995).

Managers can influence the research-practice merger through a variety of practical initiatives that include encouragement of nurses to participate in peer review of clinical practice, identifying times when nurses could assess up-to-date material and allocating a designated budget for journal subscription (Kenrick and Luker, 1996). Other strategies that managers can employ in promoting research utilisation include the provision of support for continuing education in research awareness, support for the formation of research interest groups and journal clubs, support for the formation of Nurse Practice Development Units, and the incorporation of research application into performance review (McKenna, 1995). The establishment of Nursing Development Units (NDUs), in which nurses develop and share a philosophy of care that includes a commitment to evidence-based practice, is a very concrete way of bringing research and practice closer together. Nurse managers have a crucial role as champions and facilitators of the establishment of NDUs (Shaw and Bosanquet, 1993).

The Role of the Nurse Educator

The role of the nurse educator in promoting research utilisation is related to the role of education in promoting research awareness, research-mindedness and the skills and intellectual capacities for research utilisation. Of particular importance is the need to develop the nurse's ability to make competent critical evaluations of research studies and to assess their utility in practice (Closs and Cheater, 1994).

Educators need to be clear about the overall aim of the research element of the curriculum (Clark and Sleep, 1991). They need to consider the relationship between teaching strategies and research-related learning outcomes. The important consideration for educators is 'what to teach?' and 'how to teach it?' (Kramer et al., 1981). In this regard, a distinction is made between 'teaching research' and 'research teaching'. Teaching research is concerned with teaching about the procedural aspects of the research process and generally involves developing knowledge and skills related to reading and conducting research. Research teaching, on the other hand, involves the use of research findings in teaching content, in which educators incorporate research evidence into both theoretical and clinical teaching inputs (Closs and Cheater, 1994; Clark and Sleep, 1991). It involves educators making explicit connections between recommended nursing practices and the knowledge base from which these recommendations are drawn, and in this way, exposing the learner to research evidence at all stages of the curricular process (Rees, 1992). Advocating research teaching over the teaching research approach, Downs (1998: 247) comments: 'Research in nursing needs to be released from the jailhouse of special courses and become the base from which all clinical teaching proceeds'.

The Role of the Individual Practitioner

While it is argued that individual practitioners alone are not in a position to achieve research utilisation, it is they who will ultimately be required to effect the practice changes suggested by research. Indeed practitioners themselves may be in a position to identify clinical problems that may be brought to the attention of researchers (McKenna, 1995). The practitioner has a role in generating researchable problems, through questioning of practices and procedures. While most practitioners are not expected to conduct research, all practitioners have a professional responsibility to question their practices in the light of research. In this sense, practitioners can be the originators and the real owners of those clinical problems that require examination through research.

Achieving Research Utilisation Through Systematic Reviews, Meta-Analysis and Clinical Guidelines

The utilisation of research requires that the available research evidence is gathered, reviewed, critically analysed and evaluated in terms of its scientific merit and applicability. The process of conducting this work is a systematic or integrative review of literature and the goal of such a review is to provide a ready synthesis of research knowledge from multiple studies (Mead, 1996). Systematic reviews involve systematically locating, appraising and synthesising research evidence from a variety of research studies, in order to obtain a reliable overview of the evidence to date (Droogan and Song, 1996). They represent a research–use strategy with which nurses can develop scientifically based nursing practice guidelines for immediate use by the reader (Beyea and Nicoll, 1995). Such reviews are an increasingly available means of informing practitioners about the research evidence related to the effectiveness of nursing interventions and, as such, represent an important means of ensuring evidence-based practice (Droogan and Song, 1996). Many systematic reviews are available on the Internet and in CD-ROM format, and include such databases as the Cochran Library and the Database of Abstracts of Reviews of Effectiveness (DARE) (Droogan and Song, 1996). The National Health Service Centre for Reviews and Dissemination also publishes systematic reviews (Mead, 1996).

A means of synthesising all the available evidence on a given aspect of practice into a single area of knowledge is meta-analysis (Mead, 1996). Meta-analysis is a form of research on research, involving synthesis of the results of numerous studies (Parahoo, 1997). Meta-analysis may be undertaken as part of a systematic review and involves the application of statistical analysis to the outcomes of multiple studies, producing a combined overall picture of the evidence related to a particular area. Decisions about which studies to include in a meta-analysis exercise are based on consideration of such factors as the context, the study population, the nature of the intervention and the reported outcomes (Greener and Grimshaw, 1996). Meta-analysis may produce combined findings that generate more robust evidence than traditional reviews of literature (Greener and Grimshaw, 1996).

Clinical guidelines are a means by which practice can be evaluated and are statements that are designed to assist the delivery of quality care (Von Degenberg, 1996). They may be developed from a number of sources, including the views of expert practitioners, systematic reviews of literature, or combinations of these sources (Dickson, 1996). From systematic reviews, it is possible to present clinical guidelines in the form of clinical handbooks for nurses to use in their everyday practice (Williams et al., 1997).

MODELS OF RESEARCH UTILISATION

Nursing scholars have long recognised the complexity of research utilisation. Numerous attempts at understanding the nature of the research utilisation process have been undertaken, and have resulted in the publication of a variety of models, which seek to characterise the process in theoretical and practical terms. These research utilisation models are both descriptive and prescriptive in nature, are based on a number of research utilisation initiatives, and they point to the barriers and facilitators of research utilisation (White et al., 1995).

Three Research Utilisation Models

The Conduct and Utilisation of Research in Nursing (CURN) Project was a research utilisation initiative, undertaken by the Michigan Nurses Association, that was aimed at promoting the conduct of clinical research and at translating research findings into practice (Horsley et al., 1983). Within the CURN model, research utilisation is viewed as an organisational process, involving a series of organisational functions including the identification and synthesis of multiple validated and replicated studies, the transfer of this knowledge into clinical protocols, and the implementation and evaluation of these protocols in practice (White et al., 1995). Organisational commitment and an organisational climate supportive of change are regarded as being essential to the attainment of research utilisation (Horsley et al., 1983).

The Stetler model of research utilisation (Stetler et al., 1995) envisages a practitioner-oriented perspective in research utilisation (Mitchell,

1994). This model requires that individuals or organisations critically address the issues of the scientific soundness of the relevant studies, the desirability and feasibility of applying findings to a specific nursing situation and the level of application warranted (White et al., 1995). The model proposes a utilisation process in which the practitioner is required to review and critique research in terms of its scientific validity and its fit and feasibility for the targeted practice situation. The practitioner selects the type and nature of use or non-use of the reviewed findings, translates multiple applicable findings into specific details for practice and evaluates the outcomes in the light of objectives established at the beginning of the process (Stetler et al., 1995). The Stetler model upholds the role of the individual practitioner in research utilisation and seeks to establish research utilisation as an integral part of the individual practitioner's everyday practice in relation to routine decision making and problem solving (White et al., 1995). It also seeks to promote critical thinking in decision making (Stetler, 1994).

The Iowa model of research utilisation was developed as '. . . a pragmatic approach to infusing research into practice' at the University of Iowa Hospitals and Clinics in North America (Titler et al., 1994: 307). The model assumes that there are several factors, called 'triggers', which encourage nurses to think about their practice and to question the rationale for their actions. These factors are identified as being of two principal types, namely 'problem-focused triggers' and 'knowledge-focused triggers'. Problem-focused triggers include those problems that are repeatedly encountered in clinical practice, or that emerge out of quality improvement programmes. Knowledge-focused triggers arise from a variety of sources including research literature and practice guide-lines that are issued by agencies and organisations. These triggers act as a powerful impetus for stimulating changes in clinical practice and they can stimulate nurses to assemble, critique and evaluate research literature in order to determine if a research base exists to guide a practice change and to determine if a change is warranted. Where a sufficient research base exists, the process proceeds towards translation of the relevant aspect of this knowledge into practice. This involves a series of steps, including the selection of practice outcomes to be achieved, the design of individual or multidisciplinary interventions, and the evaluation of the interventions. Where a research base is not sufficient to guide practice, further research is conducted, or consultation with expert colleagues is undertaken in order to illuminate the problem. Having evaluated the clinical outcomes of the intervention, a decision is made as to whether the change is appropriate for adoption in practice. Once the change has been adopted, further monitoring is required in relation to patient outcomes, effects on staff and fiscal outcomes (Titler et al., 1994).

This research utilisation model, like the CURN model, envisages research utilisation as an organisational change process, and, like the Stetler model, the Iowa model upholds the value of critical thinking in the research utilisation process (White et al., 1995). Titler et al. (1994) have reported that the adoption of the model challenges nurses to think critically about their practice and to become active participants in the conduct and use of research. Despite cultural differences, the Iowa model is suitable for adaptation outside the United States, since research utilisation requires organisational change that needs to be guided, supported and managed (Meehan, 1998). Titler et al. (1994) note that research utilisation is more likely to be successful if staff are empowered with ownership of the change.

Action Research as a Research Utilisation Model

Practitioners will more readily relate to research that addresses problems arising out of their own practice area, and the success of research utilisation is partly contingent upon the ability of research to meet the needs of practitioners (Kitson et al., 1996). Research utilisation will be more likely to occur if practitioners own the clinical problems that research addresses. Action research provides nurses with such ownership of research (Nolan and Grant, 1993). As a method that is specifically designed to bridge the gap between theory, research and practice, action research offers a compelling method for nursing (Holter and Schwartz-Barcott, 1993).

Action research is a paradigm of research that has its origins in the work of Kurt Lewin, who advocated joint studies between researchers and practitioners as a means of dealing with practical problems and proposed a four-stage process of planning, acting, observing and reflecting (Meyer, 1993). Action research is also based on critical research, which upholds the belief that research should not be an esoteric activity undertaken by researchers in isolation of the people they are studying (Webb, 1989). Rather it should be conducted as a collaborative enterprise in which researcher and practitioner identify a practice problem, use research methods to assess the problem, plan and implement change and evaluate the outcome (Parahoo, 1997). It is also based on the view that research-based knowledge should be situational and context-specific (Nolan and Grant, 1993).

Action research draws upon notions of democratic participation, professional accountability and on the critical social science notion of empowering individuals and groups (Hart and Bond, 1996). It rejects the assumption that only academics are the generators of knowledge and it upholds the practitioner as researcher. In this way, it promotes a non–elitist approach, in which practitioners themselves carry out small–scale research projects (Rolfe, 1996). Research is done *with* and *for* people and not *on* them (Meyer, 1993). Action research also assumes that practitioners are best placed to interpret the findings of research and turn these findings into actions that are most likely to benefit their patients (Rolfe, 1996).

As a practical enterprise, action research has been described as a cyclical process involving situational analysis and problem identification, design of an action plan, implementation and evaluation of the action and decision making about future action, based upon reflection on the action (McKiernan, 1992). As a cyclical process, each action cycle may be repeated until such time as practitioners and researchers are satisfied that the practice problem has been addressed in the fullest possible way (Figure 1).

Figure 1. Action research model (adapted from McKiernan, 1992)

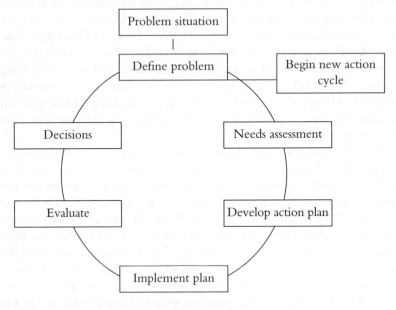

In a single action cycle, researcher and practitioners analyse the practice situation that has given rise to the perceived need for action by collecting data using quantitative and/or qualitative methods. Data are then analysed in the light of research literature, so that the local situation is understood more fully, and a shared perception of the problem is established between researcher and practitioners (Nolan and Grant, 1993). This mutually shared understanding enhances the validity of the findings (Parahoo, 1997) and gives the action strategy its focus. An action strategy is then planned that will seek to address the problem, and during the phase of implementation, there is close monitoring of the effects of the change. On completion of the implementation or action phase, there follows a phase of evaluation and reflection, in which the new practice situation is studied and the original problem restated. There is reflection on the changes that have taken place and any further changes that are needed are considered. At this point a new action cycle can begin.

Action research is characterised by its concern to solve practical problems and to bring about change. Unlike much other research, which produces knowledge that may take many years between its generation and its application, action research is concerned with the 'here and now' (Parahoo, 1997). For these reasons, it is proposed as an alternative model of research utilisation in that it represents a means by which practitioners can identify and attempt to solve local, specific practice problems. As a context-specific model, it depends on the knowledge that is generated and owned by practitioners themselves. The practitioner, as researcher, retains control and direction over the implementation of the research knowledge (Rolfe, 1994). Knowledge application is more likely to occur on this basis.

SUMMARY AND CONCLUSIONS

This chapter has examined the theoretical and practical aspects of research utilisation. In pointing to evidence that suggests that much clinical practice remains uninfluenced by relevant research, the chapter explored some of the factors which act as barriers and facilitators of research utilisation. All those engaged either directly or indirectly in clinical care have roles and responsibilities in relation to research utilisation, including clinicians, researchers, educators and nurse managers.

Research utilisation models exist to aid our understanding of the research utilisation process and they offer a framework for those deliberately engaged in practice innovation and development. Research utilisation is a complex process that requires consideration of the idiosyncrasies of the particular, including local patterns of practice, historical and cultural differences, as well as contextual factors, such as the levels of human and material resources.

REFERENCES

Alderton, J. (1983) Responsibility for research, *Nursing Times*, 79 (23): 56–7.

Beyea, S. C. and Nicoll, L. H. (1995) Administration of injections via the intramuscular route: an integrative review of the literature and research-based protocol for the procedure, *Applied Nursing Research*, 8 (1): 23–33.

Bircumshaw, D. (1990) The utilization of research findings in clinical nursing practice, *Journal of Advanced Nursing*, 15: 1272–80.

Brett, J. L. L. (1987) Use of nursing practice research findings, *Nursing Research*, 36 (6): 344–9.

Camiah, S. (1997) Utilisation of research in practice and application strategies to raise research awareness amongst nurse practitioners: a model for success, *Journal of Advanced Nursing*, 26: 1193–202.

Carter, D. (1996) Barriers to the implementation of research findings in practice, *Nurse Researcher*, 4 (2): 30–40.

Champion, V. L. and Leach, A. (1989) Variables related to research utilisation in nursing: an empirical investigation, *Journal of Advanced Nursing*, 14: 705–10.

Clark, H. C. and Sleep, J. (1991) The what and how of teaching research, *Nurse Education Today*, 11: 172–8.

Closs, S. J. and Cheater F. M. (1994) Utilisation of nursing research: culture, interest and support, *Journal of Advanced Nursing*, 19: 762–73.

Deacon, L. (1986) Pressure sores: does anyone read research? *Nursing Times*, 82 (32), suppl.: 57–9.

Dickson, R. (1996) Developing guidelines for clinical practice, *Nurse Researcher*, 4 (1): 5–14.

Downs, F. S. (1998) The rightful place of research in academia, *Nursing Outlook*, 46 (5): 246–7.

Droogan, J. and Song, F. (1996) The process and importance of systematic reviews, *Nurse Researcher*, 4 (1): 15–26.

Dunn, V., Crichton, N., Roe, B., Seers, K., and Williams, K. (1998) Using research for practice: a UK experience of the BARRIERS scale, *Journal of Advanced Nursing*, 12: 1203–10.

Edwards-Beckett, J. (1990) Nursing research utilisation techniques, *Journal of Nursing Administration*, 20 (11): 887–95.

Goode, C. J., Butcher, L. A., Cipperley, J. A., Ekstrom, J., Gosch, B. A., Hayes, J. E., Lovett, M. K., and Welldorf, S. A. (1991) *Research Utilisation: A Study Guide*. Ida Grove, Iowa: Horne Video Productions.

Government of Ireland (1998) *Report of the Commission on Nursing: A Blueprint for the Future*. Dublin: Government Publications.

Greener, J. and Grimshaw, J. (1996) Using meta-analysis to summarise evidence within systematic reviews, *Nurse Researcher*, 4 (1): 27–38.

Griffith, D. (1987) Ritual pursuits, *Nursing Times*, 83 (4): 68.

Hancock, C. (1993) Promoting nursing research: the RCN role, *Nurse Researcher*, 1 (2): 72–80.

Hart, E. and Bond, M. (1996) Making sense of action research through the use of a typology, *Journal of Advanced Nursing*, 23: 152–9.

Hefferin, E, Horsley, J., and Ventura, M. (1982) Promoting research based nursing: the nurse administrator's role, *Journal of Nursing Administration*, 12: 4–41.

Hicks, C. (1997) The dilemma of incorporating research into clinical practice, *British Journal of Nursing*, 6 (9): 511–15.

Holter, I. M. and Schwartz-Barcott, D. (1993) Action research: What is it? How has it been used and how can it be used in nursing? *Journal of Advanced Nursing*, 18: 298–304.

Horsley, J. A., Crane, J., Crantree, M. K., and Wood, D. J. (1983) *Using Research to Improve Practice: A Guide*. Philadelphia: W.B. Saunders.

Humphris, D. (1997) Implementing research findings in practice, *Nursing Standard*, 11 (33): 49–54.

Hunt, J. M. (1996) Barriers to research utilisation, *Journal of Advanced Nursing*, 23: 423–5.

Hunt, M. (1987) The process of translating research findings into practice, *Journal of Advanced Nursing*, 12: 101–10.

Kenrick, M. and Luker, K. A. (1996) An exploration of the influence of managerial factors on research utilisation in district nursing practice, *Journal of Advanced Nursing*, 23: 697–704.

Kevelighan, H. (1994) Research utilisation by nurses using continence promotion as a case study. Unpublished Master of Medical Science (in Nursing) thesis. National University of Ireland.

Kitson, A. (1997) Using evidence to demonstrate the value of nursing, *Nursing Standard*, 11 (28): 34–9.

Kitson, A., Ahmed, L. B., Harvey, G., Seers, K., and Thompson, D. R. (1996) From research to practice: one organisational model for promoting research-based practice, *Journal of Advanced Nursing*, 23: 430–40.

Kramer, M., Holaday, B. and Hoeffer, B. (1981) The teaching of nursing research – Part II: A literature review of teaching strategies, *Nurse Educator*, March–April: 30–7.

Lacey, E. A. (1994) Research utilisation in nursing practice: a pilot study, *Journal of Advanced Nursing*, 19: 987–95.

MacGuire, J. M. (1990) Putting nursing research findings into practice: research utilisation as an aspect of the management of change, *Journal of Advanced Nursing*, 15: 414–620.

McKenna, H. P. (1995) Dissemination and application of research findings: some problems and possible solutions, in: *Nursing Research: Luxury or Necessity for Practice: Proceedings of An Bord Altranais National Conference*, Dublin, 23 November 1995, Dublin: An Bord Altranais.

McKiernan, J. (1992) *Curriculum Action Research*. Dublin: Kogan Page.

Mead, D. (1996) Using nursing initiatives to encourage the use of research, *Nursing Standard*, 10 (19): 33–6.

Meehan, T. (1997) *Research Appreciation*. Dublin: National Distance Education Centre.

Meehan, T. (1998) Evidence based practice, *Quality Assurance in Nursing Update*, 4 (2).

Meyer, J. E. (1993) New paradigm research in practice: the trials and tribulations of action research, *Journal of Advanced Nursing*, 18: 1066–72.

Miller, J. and Messenger, S. (1978) Obstacles to applying nursing research findings, *American Journal of Nursing*, 78 (4): 632–6.

Mitchell, C. A. (1994) The evolution of research: from science to practice, in: G. LoBiondo-Wood and J. Haber (eds), *Nursing Research: Methods, Critical Appraisal and Utilisation*. St Louis: Mosby: 55–87.

Murray, Y. (1988) Tradition rather than cure, *Nursing Times*, 84 (38): 75, 79–80.

Myco, F. (1980) Nursing research information: are nurse educators and practitioners seeking it out? *Journal of Advanced Nursing*, 5: 637–46.

Nolan, M. and Grant, G. (1993) Action research and quality of care: a mechanism for agreeing basic values as a precursor to change, *Journal of Advanced Nursing*, 18: 305–11.

Parahoo, K. (1998) Research utilisation and research-related activities of nurses in Northern Ireland, *International Journal of Nursing Studies*, 35: 283–91.

Parahoo, K. (1997) *Nursing Research: Principles, Process and Issues*. London: Macmillan.

Polit, D. F. and Hungler, B. P. (1995) *Nursing Research: Principles and Methods* (5th edn). Philadelphia: J. B. Lippincott.

Rees, C. (1992) Practising research-based teaching, *Nursing Times*, 8 (88): 55.

Rodgers, S. (1994) An exploratory study of research utilisation by nurses in general medical and surgical wards, *Journal of Advanced Nursing*, 20: 904–11.

Rolfe, G. (1994) Towards a new model of nursing research, *Journal of Advanced Nursing*, 19: 969–75.

Rolfe, G. (1996) Going to extremes: action research, grounded practice and the theory-practice gap in nursing, *Journal of Advanced Nursing*, 24: 1315–20.

Shaw, J. T. and Bosanquet, N. (1993) *Nursing Development Units: A Way to Develop Nurses and Nursing*. London: King's Fund Centre.

Stetler, C. B. (1994) Refinement of the Stetler/Marram model for application of research findings to practice, *Nursing Outlook*, 42 (1): 15–25.

Stetler, C. B., Baustita, C., Vernale-Hannon, C., and Foster, J. (1995) Enhancing research utilisation by clinical nurse specialists, *Nursing Clinics of North America*, 30 (3), 457–68.

Titler, M. G., Kleiber, C., Steelman, V., Goode, C., Rakel, B., Barry-Walker, I., Small, S., and Buckwalter, K. (1994) Infusing research into practice to promote quality care, *Nursing Research*, 43 (5): 307–13.

Von Degenberg, K. (1996) Clinical guidelines: improving practice at local level, *Nursing Standard*, 10 (19): 37–9.

Webb, C. (1989) Action research: philosophy, methods and personal experience, *Journal of Advanced Nursing*, 14: 403–10.

Webb, C. and McKenzie, J. (1993) Where are we now? Research-mindedness in the 1990s, *Journal of Clinical Nursing*, 2: 129–33.

White, J. M., Leske, J. S. and Pearcy, J. M. (1995) Models and processes of research utilisation, *Nursing Clinics of North America*, 30 (3): 409–20.

Williams, K. S., Crichton, N. J. and Roe, B. (1997) Disseminating research evidence: a controlled trial in continence care, *Journal of Advanced Nursing*, 25: 691–8.

7
Ethical Issues in Research

Abbey Hyde and Margaret P. Treacy

Virtually every book on nursing research, and every student thesis or dissertation on nursing contains a chapter or section on the issue of ethical dimensions in research, and the inclusion of the present chapter suggests that this book is no different. Attention to ethical issues in research is considered so central to the research process that some nursing journals refuse to publish work where access to a study population has by-passed an ethics committee, regardless of whether or not respondents were in danger of being harmed or how inspiring the findings might be. A consciousness by researchers of the need to satisfy the research community that the highest ethical standards have been maintained has led to squeaky clean accounts in nursing publications of the steps taken to ensure adherence to accepted ethical guidelines and principles. However, experienced researchers know that any understanding reached between the researcher and participant about the nature of the research is mediated by factors that pervade written guidelines or principles that might exist. This arises because human interactions in the research process are often complex, unpredictable and fluid.

In this chapter, a critical account of the procedures and practices of ethics in nursing research is presented. Following an exploration of established bases for ethical decision making, the proliferation of protections constructed to safeguard research subjects, such as ethical guidelines and ethics committees, are reviewed. The implementation and operations of some of these insulating strategies and difficulties that might arise in practice are then considered. The chapter elucidates the delicate balance between inflexibility in ethical rule-following and the need for safeguards that surpass sole reliance on the integrity of the researcher.

MAKING ETHICAL DECISIONS

In Ireland, nurses' responsibility when undertaking research is indicated in An Bord Altranais's *Code for Professional Conduct for Each Nurse and Midwife* (An Bord Altranais, 1988) as follows:

> In taking part in research, the principles of confidentiality and the provision of appropriate information to enable an informed judgement to be made by the patient must be safeguarded. The nurse has an obligation to ascertain that the research is sanctioned by the appropriate body and to ensure that the rights of the patient are protected at all times. The nurse should be aware of ethical policies and procedures in his/her area of practice.

Underpinning this statement and the requirements and safeguards therein are a number of complex ethical principles, which are the basis of practical decisions and judgements both in nursing care and in nursing research.

Philosophers have long attempted to identify a basis for ethical decision making. Beauchamp and Childress (1989: 6) state that, when considering if a judgement is morally correct, what is really being considered is 'which judgement has the strongest moral reasons behind it . . .'. They highlight the need for transparency with regard to the ethical principles underpinning ethical judgements, and propose an approach to deliberation and justification with decisions 'justified by moral rules, which in turn are justified by principles, which ultimately are defended by an ethical theory' (Beauchamp and Childress, 1989: 7). Well-established principles expounded as the basis for ethical decision making are autonomy, non-maleficence, beneficence, and justice. In endeavouring to uphold these four principles, protections such as informed consent, confidentiality, and so forth have been brought to bear.

Autonomy

Autonomy refers to freedom to determine one's own actions and autonomous choices are considered central if the principle of autonomy is to be defended. Smith and Hunt (1997) point out that if an individual's autonomy is to be protected in the course of research then individuals must be free to make their own decisions regarding participation. Tunna (1997: 535) identifies four elements for consent to be valid: it must be voluntary; the person must be 'fully informed'; the person must have the capacity to make the decision; and he or she must be in a position to reject the invitation to participate. The principle of autonomy also demands that confidentiality and anonymity be protected.

Nonmaleficence

Nonmaleficence is related to the concepts of harm
due care (Beauchamp and Childress, 1989: 124). I
maxim 'first do no harm'. A related yet separate cor
(see below), which refers to the duty to care. Nonma
ficence, while associated, are not treated as one and t
do so obscures distinctions. It is suggested that that
do harm seems stronger than beneficence or 'to do g
and Childress, 1989: 122). Harm may be emotional or   and the
process of engaging in research may cause emotional distress (Smith and
Hunt, 1997). Smith and Hunt (1997) point out that 'doing no harm'
demands that a standard of care be established.

Beneficence

Beneficence relates to the more positive concept of contributing to the
welfare of others. It is noted that beneficence may involve a professional
in manipulating the truth if he/she considers it to be in a client's best
interests (Beauchamp and Childress, 1989). However, acting in the
client's best interest represents paternalism in that those who 'know
better' control the flow of information to and make decisions for others.
There is obvious potential for paternalism to conflict with the principle
of autonomy (Beauchamp and Childress, 1989). Beauchamp and Childress
(1989: 247) suggest that paternalistic interventions must always be justified
and 'the balance seldom allows beneficence to override respect for autonomy'. It is also suggested that the researcher has a responsibility to act in
a positive way to protect participants, and this principle almost places the
researcher in a watchguard role for the subject (Smith and Hunt, 1997).

Justice

While numerous theories of justice exist, each highlights a material
principle that is important for moral reflection on issues of justice and
health policy. The principle of justice requires that people should be
dealt with in a fair way; however, it also involves an element of what an
individual deserves (Beauchamp and Childress, 1989). Consequently
justice is described as a complex principle. Smith and Hunt (1997: 242)
state that the principle implies that '[i]ndividuals will be treated therefore
in proportion to their standing' in a given society and they suggest that
this is a difficult concept because it implies that all people are not valued
to the same degree in society. They further point out that on this basis
resources can be allocated in relation to need or merit. In terms of

n this is a complex principle because individuals may be included deed excluded from studies by virtue of the position they hold in ociety. Beauchamp and Childress (1989: 259) suggest that the principle of formal justice states that people must be treated equally in spite of differences unless it can be demonstrated 'that there is a difference between them relevant to the treatment at stake'.

ETHICAL GUIDELINES AND PROCEDURES

Nurse researchers have a number of sources available to them that provide guidelines on how to embrace the above principles in their research practice. Beyond the discipline of nursing, generic ethical criteria exist upon which nursing research may be guided; these criteria usually have their origins in medical research. Specific to nursing research, in addition to An Bord Altranais guidelines referred to earlier, other nursing bodies at national and international levels have published codes for appropriate ethical conduct. Researchers can also access ethical guidelines and knowledge of their practical application through nursing research texts (Holloway and Wheeler, 1996; Polit and Hungler, 1995; LoBiondo-Wood and Haber, 1994; Smith and Hunt, 1997; Parahoo, 1997; Burns and Grove, 1997). A common (and increasingly mandatory) procedure for monitoring the implementation of these guidelines is through a third party in the form of an ethics committee, which has the remit of scrutinising the proposed ethical aspects of the research.

Codes of Ethics for Research

Codes specifically designed for the protection of research subjects have sometimes been developed as it became clear that ethical principles were being violated. For example, the Nuremberg Code was developed after the Second World War when war atrocities were to be defended as medical research (Katz, 1972, cited in LoBiondo-Wood and Haber, 1994). This code encapsulates ten articles for the protection of research subjects.[1] Since then the World Medical Association produced the Declaration of Helsinki (World Medical Association, 1964, amended 1975, 1983, 1989)[2] which focuses on informed consent and the subject's best interest. In the USA, The National Commission for the Protection of Human Subjects of Biomedical and Behavioural Research was established in 1974. It identified the principles of respect, beneficence and justice as important when conducting research on human subjects (Burns and Grove, 1997). The Department of Health and Human Services (DHHS) in the USA subsequently published regulations for the conduct of research. These regulations addressed essentials for informed consent, documentation, membership of Institutional Review Boards, and exempted and expedited review boards for certain kinds of research. They also addressed criteria for Institutional Review Board approval of research (Department of Health and Human Services, 1983, 1991 cited in Burns and Grove, 1997: 199–200).

Within nursing, ethical principles and codes have been developed by, among others, the Royal College of Nursing (RCN) in the United Kingdom and the International Council of Nurses (ICN) (Royal College of Nursing, 1993; International Council of Nurses, 1996).

The RCN identifies seven ethical principles to protect subjects and bases ethical guidelines for the conduct of research on these principles. These principles and a brief interpretation are summarised in Figure 1.

Figure 1. Seven Ethical Principles to Protect Subjects of Research

1 *Beneficence* – doing good to people

2 *Nonmaleficence* – not harming people

3 *Fidelity* – a relationship based on trust; clients entrust themselves to the care of nurses

4 *Justice* – being fair

5 *Autonomy* – respecting people as autonomous persons; not unjustly exploiting relationships that are unequal

6 *Veracity/honesty and informed consent* – potential subjects' decisions to take part of their own free will in research means that they must be given accurate and clear information

7 *Confidentiality* – the protection of information related to participants that is gleaned in the course of research

Source: Royal College of Nursing (1993) *Ethical Principles for Protection of Subjects*

The Royal College of Nursing guidelines point out that confidentiality is also a central issue in the development of trust, respecting the principles of justice, nonmaleficence and autonomy. Based on these principles the RCN has drawn up ethical guidelines for nursing research (Royal College of Nursing, 1993). Areas covered in the guidelines include the integrity of the researcher, responsibility to subjects, and relations with relevant others such as sponsors and so forth. It notes that information about a study and a participant's role in it should always be given in writing and that participant's consent should always be recorded whether written or verbal. What is emphasised in the guidelines is that consent must be informed. In addition it states that where human subjects are to be part of a study, approval must be sought from 'an appropriate research ethics committee' (Royal College of Nursing, 1993: 13). Also covered are guidelines for nurses in senior positions where research is undertaken and for nurses practising in such settings (Royal College of Nursing, 1993). The former are advised of the need to ensure that the research is relevant, that procedures for the voluntary consent of subjects are in place, and that promises of anonymity and confidentiality of subjects are respected. Practitioners are advised to understand the principle of informed consent and to ensure that the research is carried out in an 'ethically acceptable way'. As data collectors, especially where they occupy a dual role, the practitioner's role in confidentiality is emphasised. Data collected for research purposes cannot be referred to in the course of other work, and data gathered in the course of a nursing work role cannot be made available to the research team unless prior agreement is reached on this.

The principles reflected in the RCN (1993) guidelines are also reflected in the guidelines published by the International Council of Nurses (1996). For individuals considering participating in research, the ICN assimilates the principles into four rights: the right not to be harmed, the right of full disclosure, the right of self-determination and the right of privacy, anonymity and confidentiality (International Council of Nurses, 1996: 7–8).

While the same principles are at the basis of all the aforementioned guidelines, some differences in interpretation may be noted. For example the ICN (1996: 12) suggests, among other things, that written consent must always be obtained from subjects whereas the RCN (1993: 12) guidelines indicate that consent, while it must be recorded, may be written or verbal.

Guidelines on Ethical Conduct for Research in Nursing Texts

The rather crude guidelines provided in codes of ethics like those referred to above require further clarification for potential nurse researchers, and nursing research textbooks are a useful source for such elaboration. However, suggestions offered by authoritative sources in nursing texts are by no means unanimous in their proposals for proper ethical conduct. While some literature recommends written informed consent as standard practice (Young Brockopp and Hastings-Tolsma, 1995; see also Meehan, chapter 5), others are more flexible in their approach. For example, Burns and Grove (1997: 213) discuss circumstances in which written consent may be waived and cite the Department of Health and Human Services (1991) regulations as follows:

Written consent may be waived in research that 'presents no more than minimal risk of harm to subjects and involves no procedures for which written consent is normally required outside of the research context'.

In such instances it is suggested that completion of a research questionnaire may be used as an indication of consent (Burns and Grove, 1997: 213). Burns and Grove (1997) also point out that written consent may also be waived where 'the only record linking the subject and the research would be the consent document and the principal risk would be potential harm resulting from a breach of confidentiality. Each subject will be asked whether the subject wants documentation linking the subject with the research, and the subject's wishes will govern' (Department of Health and Human Services, 1983 cited in Burns and Grove, 1997: 213). Regardless of 'whether written consent is waived or required' they assert that all elements of consent must be covered (Burns and Grove, 1997: 213). An aspect of informed consent, which appears to be unanimously expressed in guidelines, is the need for all potential research subjects to be given a written explanation regarding the research.

LoBiondo-Wood and Haber (1994: 323) suggest that written consent is appropriate but acknowledge that most researchers 'obtain consent through personal discussion with potential subjects'. If the risk to participants is minimal, they propose that the researcher may simply have to provide participants with a verbal account of the study and an explanation; sometimes the completion and return of questionnaires may be sufficient evidence of informed consent. In such instances LoBiondo-Wood and Haber (1994) recommend that the Institutional Review Board, which must approve all research proposals, be asked to advise on such exceptions.[3]

Ethics Committees

It is widely asserted in literature on research ethics that proposed research should be approved by ethics committees to ensure that ethical guidelines are adhered to in the proposed study (Baldwin, 1994; Young Brockopp and Hastings-Tolsma, 1995). Further evidence of the respectable status of such committees comes from the fact that some nursing journals reject articles for publication if the study did not received approval from a local or hospital research ethics committee (Heenan, 1995). In Britain, approval from the local research ethical committee (LREC) is mandatory if research is being carried out with National Health Service (NHS) clients or on NHS premises (Baldwin 1994; Tierney, 1995).

In Ireland, the health service does not have a blanket policy on the existence of ethics committees, although most large hospitals have such committees. These committees in some instances are set up to review particular types of research, for example randomised controlled trials. In the case of approval and access for nursing research, this may or may not be approved directly by an ethics committee. At the present time in Ireland, all initial approaches are made through the directors of nursing or of midwifery services (in many instances, these directors sit on hospital ethics' committees). Initial submissions include a research proposal outlining all aspects of the proposed work, background information on the researcher and other relevant information. The director of service negotiates access within the institution, advises on any other steps to be taken and responds to the application. Such research submissions do not always involve patients. Should research involve patients the physician in charge of the patient's treatment is also approached for permission to begin the process of recruiting participants for the study. Individual informed consent subsequently becomes the responsibility of and is negotiated by the researcher. The Medical Council (in Ireland) suggests that written consent be obtained from all participants in clinical trials. The Council advises that research committees be established in institutions where research is carried out and advises medical practitioners to channel research activities through the committee (Medical Council, 1998).

ETHICAL DIMENSIONS OF RESEARCH IN PRACTICE – SOME PRACTICAL PROBLEMS

While the various ethical guidelines outlined above provide researchers with an indication as to how to proceed, in the actual practice of research many researchers have found themselves in circumstances where adhering to these guidelines presented difficulties and dilemmas. The two most frequently recurring problem areas are related to informed consent and confidentiality.

The Practice of Informed Consent

While the components of informed consent have been detailed in research textbooks, and accounts have been written to assist would-be researchers in ensuring that the consent they might receive is given freely and willingly (Erlen, 1994), Clarke (1996) notes that merely requesting consent does not imply that potential respondents know to what they are consenting. In the past, explanations of research designs have been misunderstood by participants (Clarke, 1996). Merrell and Williams (1994) also suggest that the degree to which participants have the capacity to absorb information imparted by the researcher, both verbally and in writing at the outset of a study, is questionable. They supply an example of a study where over half the participants were unaware that they were research subjects even though they had been presented with and signed a consent form. As Tunna (1997) notes, a patient's signature on a consent form does not mean that he or she fully understands what has been agreed nor the impact his or her participation may have on him or her; there is more to valid consent than a signature on a piece of paper.

It has also been argued that all research is to some extent secret, given that it is impossible to reveal all aspects of a research project to potential participants (Roth, 1970 cited in Merrell and Williams, 1994; Clarke, 1996). Ethical guidelines (as indicated above) rarely acknowledge this, probably because to do so would allow too much leeway to individual researchers.

The method of observation has long been identified as problematic in relation to obtaining informed consent. Studies have been conducted where researchers have remained completely undercover as in Knight's and Field's (1981) study of dying patients in a British surgical ward (in this case one of the researchers passed as a nurses' aide and interactants were completely unaware that they were being studied). A more recent example is Clarke's (1996) study in a secure forensic psychiatric unit, where he too passed as a nursing auxiliary. Such studies are rare, possibly because journals would refuse to publish them on ethical grounds.

Merrell and Williams (1994) elucidate the difficulty of obtaining informed consent when the researcher occupies a variety of roles and enters into a variety of relationships in participant observation studies. The researcher may be a colleague and friend as well as researcher to those whom he or she encounters in the field, and when information is imparted by someone in the field, it is not clear under which of those roles that this is done. The difficulty of 'announcing one's presence as a researcher' (Merrell and Williams, 1994: 168) to new arrivals on the study field was also noted. Drawing on experiences from their own study, they highlight the difficulties they encountered in persistently reminding interactants that one was in the guise of researcher at the same time as volunteer or colleague. Such constant reminders that one was doing research tended to irritate interactants. Nonetheless, Merrell and Williams (1994) suggest that informed consent is not a single event but needs to be negotiated continually as the study progresses.

Merrell and Williams (1994) also discuss what they refer to as 'situational limitations and opportunities' of doing observation studies and the implications these have for gaining informed consent. The limitations refer to the lack of control the researcher has in determining whether and when an individual enters and departs from the field of study. Situational opportunities arose for Merrell and Williams (1994) in their study when friendships were established with informants that facilitated information exchange. However, whether this information was imparted with the understanding that it was given with consent for the research project or whether it was 'off the record' information from a friend was unclear to the researchers. This difficulty is aptly captured by Clarke (1996: 37) who posits that 'material gathered via dynamic relationships within small communities will reflect the ethics of the researcher more than abstract notions of informed consent'.

The problem of multiple roles in the practice of research and concomitant problem of informed consent is not unique to observation research. Paddison (1995) also identified the problem of multiple roles in interviewing colleagues. She acknowledges that in her study, interchange with informants after the audio recorder had been switched off yielded copious data, a large proportion of which was wasted because at specific times she did not perceive herself in a researcher role. Similarly, multiple agendas have been identified in action research[4] (Williams, 1995), where the researcher may adopt different roles in relation to those she is researching. The nature of action research lends itself to further difficulties with informed consent: action research aims to change conditions through the research process – the researcher may be unaware of the essence of the proposed change, as this unfolds in the emerging situation (Williams, 1995).

More recently, problems associated with informed consent in qualitative research have been widely noted, where not all issues for investigation are known at the outset of the study (Behi, 1995; Merrell and Williams, 1994). While this is particularly the case in grounded theory type projects (Merrell and Williams, 1994), almost all qualitative methodologies have an 'unknown in advance' component, given that they rely mainly on inductive reasoning. Considering that the use of qualitative methodologies has proliferated in nursing scholarship in recent years, the problems associated with achieving complete informed consent have escalated and are no longer confined to isolated projects.

One way of overcoming the problem to some extent is to negotiate consent continually while progressing in the project. This is not always possible, however, with some methods of data collection, such as the in-depth interview, because continual references to consent during an interview are in danger of obstructing the 'flow' and 'rapport' so lauded in this style of data collection. The usual advice is to reassure respondents at the outset that they do not have to answer questions about which they feel uncomfortable and so forth, yet many of the skills associated with interviewing are designed to develop rapport in order to gain the trust of the interviewee. At the extreme, it might be argued that using such tactical measures to gain the richest of data is unethical in that they are designed to lure respondents to reveal as much as possible, perhaps more than they had initially intended. This may threaten the principle of nonmaleficence, insofar as respondents may suffer from emotional distress as a consequence of a researcher's competence in getting to the core of their construction of reality. It is well established in the research literature that a well-designed interview guide begins with less sensitive issues to ease tension, and holds the more problematic ones until later. As Brannen (1988) notes, sensitive researchers adopt a cautious approach at the outset, and refrain from revealing all that lies in store, so as not to pre-empt the research problem or close ranks too soon on respondents' construction of things. Therein lies a dilemma for the qualitative researcher – even if he or she does know in advance the broad topics to be investigated, revealing some of these at the outset of the project would be at variance with sound research practice. At the root of this dilemma is the fact that interviewing takes place in a social context with all the complexities of human interaction, while research guidelines are often presented as de-contextualised, objective rules to be followed.

In addition to difficulties with informed consent in relation to certain methodologies, problems have also been noted with the concept in researching specific groups. Such groups include older people with dementia (Watson, 1994), children (Lowes, 1996), unconscious persons, and some individuals with learning disabilities and mental illness (Behi, 1995).

Finally, the practice of signing one's name to consent to anything is likely to be cross-cut by cultural beliefs, and potential participants who might otherwise be willing to partake in a study may retreat through a fear of being inveigled by their signature. It may be more appropriate, therefore, for the researcher to sign a statement detailing the nature of the information imparted about the study, how confidentiality would be guaranteed and so on, and giving a copy of this to the participant.

The Practice of Preserving Confidentiality

In addition to practical issues surrounding the concept of informed consent, routine guidelines on preserving confidentiality of clients have also been problematised in nursing research literature. Some research methodologies such as case studies, qualitative research and focus group research lend themselves to particular problems with maintaining confidentiality, particularly when researching sensitive issues. Even though participants may remain anonymous insofar as their names never appear with data, close attention to detail associated with these methodologies may mean that certain cues might reveal a participant's identity. This may be particularly relevant to Irish research, because of the relatively small population size in the country, the tendency for nurses to network with each other, and the propensity for people to have personal knowledge of and an interest in other people's lives.

Platzer and James (1997) note that in their qualitative research on lesbian and gay men's experiences of nursing care using the interview method, there was a sense of disquiet among participants that either their or their partners' identities might be revealed in the data. The position of the partners was of particular concern since information that interviewees gave about them was transmitted without the partners' fully informed consent.

Smith (1995) raises similar issues in relation to confidentiality and focus group interviews. While a focus group leader can take all feasible measures to maintain confidentiality when handling the revelations of group members, he or she cannot control what respondents may reveal after they leave the group. Individual group members, therefore, rely on fellow participants as much as the researcher to maintain confidentiality. Smith (1995) proposes that the researcher should alert participants to this danger.

McHaffie (1996) describes a further potential difficulty in relation to confidentiality, which can challenge the simplicity of ethical guidelines. This is where potentially deleterious information is revealed by participants, upon which the researcher might ordinarily (in another role) intervene. However, if researchers felt the urge to breach confidences on the basis of discrediting information they received that was deemed to be damaging to either the participant or others, our knowledge of the social world might be shut down through potential respondents' fears of research participation. At the same time, can a researcher stand by and do nothing when he or she possesses information that might arrest a catastrophe?

Problems with Ethics Committees

Recently, criticisms have been levelled at the functioning and limitations of ethics committees (Pollock and Tilley, 1988; Schrock, 1991; Hunt, 1992) and it is worth noting some of these criticisms before adding further reservations.

The absence of nurses from such committees (in the UK at least) has been noted (Hunt, 1992). In the current Irish situation, directors of nursing and midwifery are members of hospital ethics committees in many instances, but the strength of their numbers relative to physicians appears to vary and needs to be monitored as committees become more formalised. The numerically weak nursing presence noted by Hunt (1992) has implications for approval of projects with particular research methodologies that may be perceived to be 'unscientific' by the medical community. Tierney (1995) notes that questions on the application form tend to be constructed in terms of intervention-type medical research. McHaffie (1996) suggests that discrepancies may arise between the gatekeeper's perception of threat and that of the researcher. Others have contended that the protection of participants may not be a priority of ethics committees (Pollock and Tilley, 1988; Schrock, 1991; Hunt, 1992), with scientific and legal concerns instead taking precedence (Hunt, 1992).

In a highly informative article on the process of gaining ethical approval for her British study of the midwives' care of the mother relinquishing her baby for adoption, Mander (1992) highlights the inconsistency in responses she received from various ethics committees which acted as gatekeepers to potential participants. Of the six ethics committees she approached, three allowed access with little hesitation, while the other three declined. Mander requested that each of the committees refusing access review its decision and, following an interview, one committee that had earlier barred access rescinded; a second remained steadfast in its refusal while the third made no reply to her request. What Mander goes on to illuminate is that the grounds for refusal of access to potential participants by ethics committees were later refuted by the evidence she managed to procure about the sample. Among the examples she furnishes is where one ethics committee refused access on the basis that it perceived the midwife to have only a peripheral role in the process of adoption. Mander (1992: 1463) points out that subsequent data she gleaned contradicted the committee's views on the issue. She also indicates that ethics committees criticised her method of in-depth interviewing on the assumption that only structured interviews had a 'meaningful basis'.

Ethics committees have the potential to wield considerable power because of their significant role in determining which knowledge bases about the social world are created, and which are suppressed. This can, for example, have the following negative consequences:

1 Given that most ethics committees contain the usual 'pillars of society', namely, physicians (who tend to dominate), administrators, pharmacists (Baldwin, 1994) and only sometimes lay members, nurses, and/or midwives (Tierney, 1995), research topics of concern to groups which are socially isolated, marginalised, stigmatised or considered deviant may never get past the gatekeepers. Medicine has problematised particular social groups in the past, such as gays, feminists, and single mothers (Zola, 1975) and may be less favourable to spending research funds on those who challenge the establishment. Blocking off research on such individuals may reinforce their peripheral status by restricting the development of challenging discourses that present an alternative view of reality in their favour.

2 Since more and more areas of social life have been medicalised, that is, subsumed under medical jurisdiction, the number of groups and individuals to whom medicine can control access as research participants has increased. Included among the 'patient' population are older people, pregnant women, dying people, and so forth. Given that many 'normal' life processes are overlaid by medical intervention, medical personnel, in their gatekeeper role, in turn have some degree of control over more and more knowledge bases in nursing and the social sciences.

3 Ethics committees can veto studies that they do not consider to be 'scientifically' sound. The experiences of those seeking access suggest that committees have barred access to proposals with methodological strategies that were at variance with established 'science' (Mander, 1992). As Hunt (1992: 351) notes:

> The kinds of fundamental moral issues that would concern an informed public will not be raised, whatever guidelines are published and whatever laws are passed, if the biomedical paradigm and the corporate of medical goods manufacturers continue to define the very parameters of 'valid' or acceptable research in healthcare.

Newer and less conventional research methodological strategies are in danger of being thwarted with serious implications for epistemological advances in nursing and the social sciences.

4 Ethics committees can, potentially at least, operate to secure greater power for a small group of professionals leading to elitism.

The above criticisms notwithstanding, the idea of ethics committees to protect potential research subjects is, broadly speaking, a positive development. However, ethics committees themselves need to be the subject of scrutiny to ensure that their operations are inclusive, just, and egalitarian.

EVALUATING THE ETHICAL COMPONENTS OF A STUDY

Evaluating the ethical component of a study can also be highly problematic. For example, the written account of the process of obtaining informed consent in research reports cannot fully capture the intricacies of the researcher–respondent interaction, and a flawless report of how consent was obtained, documented and so forth can mask a brash, coercive style of interaction. Furthermore, pressure on researchers from a threat of study findings being rejected for publication or a thesis failing at examination on the grounds of ethical conduct is likely to encourage uncontroversial, 'safe', versions of how the ethics of a project progressed. This may occur regardless of the researcher's own doubts about the ethics of the project, which, if exposed, might in fact have demonstrated intellectual and moral maturity. Indeed, it is the experience of one of the present authors (Hyde) that thesis students frequently check first whether various (ethical) events in their research should be documented or omitted through a fear that complete honesty might damage the thesis results.

Furthermore, the dynamics involved in gaining entirely free and unbiased consent are rarely witnessed by anyone other than the two parties involved, and the implementation of guidelines as to how to avoid even gentle encouragement that might be construed as 'biased information' fall back on the integrity of the researcher. It is not being suggested here that details of informed consent and guidelines as to how to gain consent that is entirely free are useless. On the contrary, they are highly useful to the ethical conduct of research. The point is that they cannot be adequately evaluated by consumers of research reports and the wider research community because of the significant yet subtle potential gap between how researchers say they behaved and how participants constructed that behaviour.

SUMMARY AND CONCLUSION

Ethical decision making in research involves a process of deliberation, and ethical principles have become the basis of codes and guidelines in research to assist in the deliberation process. These guidelines attempt to identify rights and make suggestions as to how participants may be protected. Research ethics committees in the health services act as filters with the remit of protecting research subjects. However, the powers vested in such committees and their operations have begun to be questioned. It has also been noted in this chapter that while codes of ethical conduct provide essential safeguards for research participants, they are not incontrovertible; sound ethical conduct in research goes beyond written guidelines to draw on the integrity of the researcher. In the final analysis, it would seem that in the practice of research, ethical principles which inform the guidelines are more important than rigid rule following.

NOTES

1 Reproduced as Appendix B (International Council of Nurses, 1996).
2 Reproduced in Appendix A (International Council of Nurses, 1996).
3 Institutional Review Boards review research from the point of view of protection of subjects' rights. In the USA the National Research Act 1974 requires all grant applications involving human subjects to indicate that they have established an IRB. In other instances Research Advisory Committees may be established for similar purposes. (LoBiondo-Wood and Haber, 1994: 330).

4 Action research is a research strategy that involves collaboration between researcher and participants in identifying an area that requires change, and working together to achieve that change while at the same time continuing to monitor progress (Bowling, 1997). The process of research is cyclic with a dynamic relationship between research, practice, and evaluation (see the section on action research in chapter 6, pp. 87–9).

REFERENCES

Baldwin, J. (1994) How to gain ethical committee approval, *Modern Midwife*, 4 (11): 27–9.

Beauchamp, T.L. and Childress, J.F. (1989) *Principles of Biomedical Ethics* (3rd edn). New York/Oxford: Oxford University Press.

Behi, R. (1995) The individual's right to informed consent, *Nurse Researcher*, 3 (1): 14–23.

An Bord Altranais (1988) *The Code of Professional Conduct for Each Nurse and Midwife*. Dublin: An Bord Altranais.

Bowling, A. (1997) *Research Methods in Health: Investigating Health and Health Services*. Buckingham: Open University Press.

Brannen, J. (1988) Research note: the study of sensitive subjects, *Sociological Review*, 36 (1): 552–63.

Burns, N., and Grove, S.K. (1997) *The Practice of Nursing Research: Conduct, Critique and Utilization*. (3rd edn). Philadelphia: W.B. Saunders.

Clarke, L. (1996) Covert participant observation in a secure forensic unit, *Nursing Times*, 27 (48): 37–40.

Department of Health and Human Services (1983) *Protection of Human Subjects*. Code of Federal Regulations, Title 45, Public Welfare, Part 46. Cited in N. Burns and S.K. Grove (1997) *The Practice of Nursing Research: Conduct, Critique and Utilization*. (3rd edn). Philadelphia: W.B. Saunders.

Department of Health and Human Services (1991) *Protection of Human Subjects*. Code of Federal Regulations, Title 45, Public Welfare, Part 46. Cited in N. Burns and S.K. Grove (1997) *The Practice of Nursing Research: Conduct, Critique and Utilization* (3rd edn). Philadelphia: W.B. Saunders.

Erlen, J.A. (1994) Informed consent: the consent component, *Orthopaedic Nursing*, 13 (4): 65–7.

Heenan, A. (1995) Research ethics, *Professional Nurse*, 10 (10): 615.

Holloway, I. and Wheeler, S. (1996) *Qualitative Research for Nurses*. Oxford: Blackwell.

Hunt, G. (1992) Local research ethics committees and nursing: a critical look. *British Journal of Nursing*, 1 (7): 349–51.

International Council of Nurses (1996) *Ethical Guidelines for Nursing Research*. Geneva: International Council of Nurses.

Knight, M. and Field, D. (1981) A silent conspiracy: coping with dying cancer patients on an acute surgical ward, *Journal of Advanced Nursing*, 6: 221–9.

LoBiondo-Wood, G. and Haber, J. (1994) *Nursing Research: Methods Critical Appraisal and Utilization* (3rd edn). St Louis: Mosby.

Lowes, L. (1996) Paediatric nursing and research ethics: is there a conflict? *Journal of Clinical Nursing*, 5: 91–7.

Mander, R. (1992) Seeking approval for research access: the gatekeeper's role in facilitating a study of the care of the relinquishing mother, *Journal of Advanced Nursing*, 17: 1460–4.

McHaffie, H. (1996) Ethics and midwifery, *Modern Midwife*, 6 (10): 34–5.

Medical Council (1998) *Guide to Ethical Conduct and Behaviour* (5th edn). Dublin: Medical Council (Ireland).

Merrell, J. and Williams, A. (1994) Participant observation and informed consent: relationships and tactical decision-making in nursing research, *Nursing Ethics*, 1 (3):163–72.

Paddison, J. (1995) Ethical issues in qualitative studies, *Modern Midwife*, 5 (5): 23–5.

Parahoo, K. (1997) *Nursing Research: Principles, Process and Issues*. Basingstoke: Macmillan.

Platzer, H. and James, T. (1997) Methodological issues conducting sensitive research on lesbian and gay men's experience of nursing care, *Journal of Advanced Nursing*, 25: 626–33.

Polit, D. and Hungler, B. (1995) *Nursing Research: Principles and Methods* (5th edn). Philadelphia: Lippincott.

Pollock, L. and Tilley, S. (1988) Submitting for approval, *Senior Nurse*, 8 (5): 24–5.

Roth, J.A. (1970) Comments on secret observation, in: W.J. Filstead (ed.), *Qualitative Methodology: Firsthand Involvement with the Social World*. Chicago: Markham: 278–80.

Royal College of Nursing (1993) *Ethics Related to Research in Nursing*. London: Research Advisory Group, Royal College of Nursing.

Schrock, R. (1991) Moral issues in nursing research, in: D. Cormack (ed.), *The Research Process in Nursing* (2nd edn). Oxford: Blackwell: 30–9.

Smith, M.W. (1995) Ethics in focus groups: a few concerns. *Qualitative Health Research*, 5 (4): 478–86.

Smith, P. and Hunt, J.M. (1997) *Research Mindedness for Practice: An Interactive Approach for Nursing and Health Care*. New York: Churchill Livingstone.

Tierney, A. (1995) The role of research ethics committees, *Nurse Researcher*, 3 (1): 43–52.

Tunna, K. (1997) Research and patient rights, *Practice Nurse*, 23 May: 531–6.

Watson, R. (1994) Practical ethical issues related to the care of elderly people with dementia, *Nursing Ethics*, 1 (3): 151–62.

Williams, A. (1995) Ethics and action research, *Nurse Researcher*, 2 (3): 49–59.

World Medical Association (1964) *Declaration of Helsinki: Recommendations Guiding Physicians in Biomedical Research Involving Human Subjects*. Adapted by the 18th World Medical Assembly, Helsinki, Finland, and June 1964. Amended by the 29th World Medical Assembly, Tokyo, Japan, October 1975; the 35th World Medical Assembly, Venice, Italy, October 1983; and the 41st World Medical Assembly, Hong Kong, September 1989. Reproduced as Appendix A in International Council of Nurses (1996) *Ethical Guidelines for Nursing Research*. Geneva: International Council of Nurses.

Young Brockopp, D. and Hastings-Tolsma, M. T. (1995) *Fundamentals of Nursing Research* (2nd edn). Boston: Jones & Bartlett.

Zola, I.K. (1975) Medicine as an institution of social control, in: C. Cox and A. Mead (eds), *Sociology of Medical Practice*. London: Macmillan: 170–85.

Part II

Application of Research Strategies

8

A Literature Review of Factors which Influence Nurses' Assessment of Pain

Kathy Redmond and Laserina O'Connor

INTRODUCTION

Pain can be controlled, in the majority of clinical situations, using relatively inexpensive and simple means (Agency for Health Care Policy and Research (AHCPR), 1993; AHCPR, 1994; World Health Organisation (WHO), 1996. Despite this fact, there is an abundance of evidence to demonstrate that a significant number of patients experience unacceptable levels of pain (Boström et al., 1997; Carr and Thomas, 1997; Zalon, 1997; Bernabei et al., 1998). This is a problem of enormous depth and scope. There is no one reason why pain is so poorly managed, indeed the problem is contributed to not only by health professionals, but also by patients, their families and the healthcare system itself (Hawthorn and Redmond, 1998).

Nurses have to make a wide range of clinical decisions about pain in their everyday clinical practice (Table 1). However, they frequently make poor clinical decisions such as underestimating the severity of a patient's pain or overestimating the effectiveness of interventions (Zalon, 1993; Stephenson, 1994; Sun and Weissman, 1994; O'Connor, 1995). Such decisions are often based upon inadequate collection and erroneous interpretation of data. A variety of factors are thought to influence the pain assessment process. These factors need to be identified, so that strategies to overcome them can be developed. Thus, the purpose of this review is to identify the factors which influence nurses' assessment of pain.

A search of the electronic databases MEDLINE and CINAHL between 1990 and 1998 was carried out. Then a handsearch of the indexes from those journals identified by the electronic search as being rich in articles on the topic was undertaken. Finally, reference lists from articles identified through the above mentioned search strategy were scanned to ensure

Table 1. Clinical Decisions Made by Nurses in Relation to Pain

- Determine the nature of the pain and its impact on the person
- Identify factors contributing to the person's expression and perception of pain
- Determine when to administer analgesic agents
- Decide what analgesic agent to administer when more than one is prescribed
- Decide what dose of analgesic to administer when a dose range is prescribed
- Determine whether the analgesic has been effective
- Determine the reasons why an intervention might not be effective
- Identify whether there is a need to change the dose, timing or type of analgesic agent and report this promptly to a physician
- Decide what non-pharmacological interventions to use

Source: Redmond (1998).

that relevant studies were not excluded. The search was limited to primary studies which had been published in English. The authors acknowledge that confining the search in this manner may mean that a significant amount of research on the subject is missing from this review and there is therefore a risk that the conclusions drawn are inaccurate or incomplete (Droogan and Cullum, 1998).

The Nature of Pain

Pain is a complex form of human suffering which spans an enormous spectrum. It varies in terms of intensity (strength or severity), quality, timing (duration and frequency of occurrence) and the amount of distress perceived and expressed by the person (Lenz et al., 1997). This is because a number of physical, psychological, social and spiritual factors influence the pain experience (Hawthorn and Redmond, 1998). For example, a person's perception and tolerance of pain can be influenced by factors such as the meaning of the pain, culture, religious beliefs, sense of control the person feels over the pain, and emotions such as anxiety and depression (Hawthorn and Redmond, 1998). Moreover, beliefs and attitudes, physiological responses, personality, gender, emotional state and the potential financial and emotional advantage associated with the pain are thought to influence pain expression (Hawthorn and Redmond,

1998). Given the subjective nature of the pain experience, the patient's self-report is the most reliable indicator of pain intensity (McCaffrey and Rolling Ferrell, 1997). However, there are many situations where patients do not express their pain verbally (Hawthorn and Redmond, 1998), and so nurses frequently have to infer pain on the basis of patients' behaviours or physiological responses. This is problematic since these are unreliable indicators of pain intensity and therefore open to misinterpretation (Sutters and Miaskowki, 1992). This highlights the complexity of the pain assessment process and how difficult it is for nurses to carry out an accurate and comprehensive assessment.

PAIN ASSESSMENT

The Nature of Assessment

Assessment is a process which has the purpose of providing the nurse with an accurate picture of a patient's current condition (Crow et al., 1995). The assessment process involves the selection, collection and organisation of pertinent clinical information which the nurse then uses to make diagnostic and management decisions (Redmond, in press). Clinical information is also collected whilst monitoring the patient and during evaluation and reassessment. Since these processes have the same overall purpose as assessment (i.e. to determine the patient's current condition), they are referred to in this chapter as assessment.

Collecting Information about Pain

Nurses collect clinical information primarily by means of interviewing, observation and measurement (Redmond, in press). Since pain is a subjective experience, interviewing patients should take precedence over the measurement of vital signs or observation of non-verbal pain expressions (McCaffrey and Rolling Ferrell, 1997). However, there are a number of factors which interfere with the collection of patients' self-reports about pain. This means that the information collected is often inadequate and the nurse is vulnerable to making erroneous clinical decisions.

Inadequate collection of patients' self-reports
There is an abundance of evidence to demonstrate that nurses do not always ask patients about their pain. For example, Paice et al. (1991) used a correlational ex post facto design to study the pain experience of randomly selected surgical oncology patients (n=34) and found that 13 (38.2 per cent) patients had never been asked about their pain. Similarly, in a quantitative study of the post-operative pain experiences of surgical

patients (n=191) it was found that nearly twenty per cent of the sample were unable to remember a nurse ever discussing their pain with them (Juhl et al., 1993). Likewise, using qualitative methodologies, Alleyne and Thomas (1994) in a study of patients with sickle cell anaemia (n=10) and Carr and Thomas (1997) in a study of post-operative patients (n=10) both reported that few of their respondents ever remembered the nurse asking them about their pain.

In two studies of patients' experience of pain in a post-operative setting, subjects stated that informal pain assessments usually coincided with the drug round or the time when the nurse was monitoring their vital signs (Carr, 1990; Carr and Thomas, 1997). Similarly, in an interview study of nurses' (n=8) assessment and priority of post surgical pain experience, many of the subjects stated that they assessed pain during their morning round or when carrying out a planned nursing activity (Boegeskov Nielsen et al., 1994). It could be argued that such timing of assessment can compromise the quality of data collected since, whilst undertaking other tasks, nurses are unlikely to place too high a priority on carrying out a comprehensive pain assessment.

Nurses may not ask patients about their pain because they experience difficulty and lack skills in communication. This was shown in a study by Wilkinson (1991) who used audio-taped recordings of assessment interviews and categorised verbal communication behaviours as either facilitative or blocking. She found that nurses use blocking behaviours in over half of their interactions with cancer patients. Although the nurses were able to identify distressing symptoms, they made little effort to elicit the intensity of each symptom or its impact on the patient. Likewise, Francke et al. (1996), in a study which employed participant observation and qualitative interviews to explore how Dutch surgical oncology nurses (n=25) cared for patients in pain, found that they carried out superficial assessments. This behaviour may reflect negative attitudes by some of the nurses about the value of carrying out comprehensive assessments. On the other hand, it may indicate that some of them felt powerless when confronted with patients in severe pain. De Schepper et al. (1997) reported similar feelings of powerlessness in a qualitative study of Dutch community nurses (n=21) who care for cancer patients with pain. Some of these nurses were reluctant to talk with patients for fear of 'stirring something up' (De Schepper et al, 1997: 425). It is important to note that these studies have been carried out in an oncology setting. Thus, it may be the cancer *per se*, as opposed to the pain, which has created the difficulties in communication, since nurses often lack confidence and do not feel competent to communicate with cancer patients, particularly those who are terminally ill (Corner and Wilson-Barnett, 1992).

Finally, patients may not be asked about their pain because nurses consider other methods of assessment as more reliable indicators of pain intensity. This was demonstrated in a survey which was distributed to nurses (n=200) attending a pain workshop (Ferrell et al., 1991). Attendees were asked to complete the questionnaire after an actual experience of caring for a patient in pain. Fifty-three (25 per cent) nurses returned the questionnaire and it was found that over half of them considered strategies such as observing the patient's activity or behaviour to be more important in assessing pain intensity than the patient's self-report. Using the vignette format, McCaffrey and Ferrell (1991) also found that over half of their sample of nurses (n=456) would select a pain rating other than the patient's self-report to assess pain intensity.

Patients' reluctance and ability to report pain
Nurses' assessment is complicated by the fact that patients are often reluctant to report pain. In a phenomenological study of the pain experience of elderly women (n=16) following surgery, Zalon (1997) found that some of the women never asked for pain medication. Others only sought medication when they experienced intolerable pain. Five women said that they endured pain because they feared becoming addicted to opioids; others tolerated pain because they believed that suffering was a woman's role. Likewise, data from in-depth qualitative interviews with surgical oncology patients (n=26) revealed that worry about addiction and other side effects of opioids was a reason for not expressing pain (Francke et al., 1996). Yates et al. (1995) carried out a series of focus group interviews with elderly nursing home patients which aimed to elicit their beliefs, attitudes and perceptions of pain management and found that patients did not report pain because they were overwhelmingly resigned to it, believing it to be an inevitable part of their illness experience or simply a feature of old age. Moreover, the subjects expressed the belief that they should not bother staff or relatives with their complaints of pain because they perceived them to be too busy or uninterested. Similar beliefs have been expressed by patients in studies carried out in a coronary care, post-operative and oncology setting (Schwartz and Keller, 1993; Francke et al., 1996; Riddell and Fitch, 1997; Carr and Thomas, 1997). It is interesting to note that nurses also perceive patients' reluctance to report pain to be a major barrier to optimal pain control (Vortherms et al., 1992; O'Brien et al., 1996; Clarke et al., 1996).

A further difficulty in the pain assessment process is that some nurses expect patients to complain spontaneously of pain, whereas it has been shown that many patients will report pain spontaneously only if it is severe (Schneider, 1987; Willetts, 1989; Hofgren et al., 1994; Mackintosh, 1994; Francke et al., 1996). Furthermore, it has been found that some

patients expect the physician or nurse to enquire about their pain or to
know that they are in pain, while others prefer the nurse to wait until
they complain of pain before initiating pain relief measures (Seers, 1987;
Carr, 1990; Winefield et al., 1990; Schwartz and Keller, 1993; Francke
and Theeuwen, 1994; Zalon, 1997; Briggs and Dean, 1998). These
findings demonstrate that patients and health professionals often hold
dichotomous expectations about how and when a patient should report
pain. Such conflicting expectations have significant potential for
compromising pain relief efforts.

Pain is a private experience which is communicated through the use
of language (Waddie, 1996). In the English language the word 'pain' is
used and interpreted in many different ways. There is ample evidence
to show that many patients do not use this word to describe a painful
symptom (Schneider 1987; Hartford et al., 1993; Francke and Theeuwen,
1994; Meehan et al., 1995). They use words such as 'heaviness',
'discomfort', 'unpleasant feeling' or 'burning' instead. Thus, if asked 'Are
you in pain?', they will answer 'No'. This demonstrates how easily break-
downs in communication can occur when nurses assume that they are
using language in the same way as their patients and highlights the
importance of nurses identifying, and thereafter using, the particular
word individual patients use to describe their pain.

Under-utilisation of pain measurement tools
Pain assessment tools provide patients with a means of expressing the
intensity of their pain and can therefore overcome some of the problems
mentioned above. However, it has been demonstrated in a number of
studies that measurement tools are still not used commonly in clinical
practice. Ferrell et al.(1991) found that 59 per cent of their sample used
a pain rating scale. This finding is commendable when compared to that
of other studies. Walker et al. (1990) administered a questionnaire to
nurses who visited patients in pain in a community setting and found
that only 18 out of 146 used a formal pain assessment tool. Similarly,
Alleyne and Thomas (1994) and Field (1996) showed that just over a
quarter of their samples had ever used a tool to assess pain. Nurses in
Francke et al.'s (1996: 36) study said it was unusual for them to use pain
assessment tools. They thought that post–operative pain was easy to
identify and therefore extensive assessment was '. . . a bit "overdone"'.
Other reasons why pain assessment charts may not be used commonly
by nurses are that they are not included routinely in the flow sheet
which documents vital signs (Scott, 1992) or simply because an easy to
administer and valid and reliable tool is not available (Nagy, 1998). In a
survey by Clarke et al. (1996), 76 per cent of the respondents reported
that they use a patient self-rating tool, although an audit of their charts

showed that only 24 per cent had evidence of the use of such self-rating tools. This does not necessarily mean that the nurses are not using pain assessment tools in practice, but the fact that they are not documenting their findings has negative implications for continuity of care and the on-going assessment of pain.

Poor documentation

Poor documentation can compromise the pain assessment process. It may lead to erroneous decision making by nurses taking over the care of a patient in pain, since they will be deprived of vital information (Camp, 1988). Even if nurses have been caring for patients for a period of time, they are still vulnerable to erroneous decision making as a result of poor documentation. This is because some will not remember information about a patient's pain accurately and others will forget it completely (Dillon McDonald, 1996).

Unfortunately, the documentation of pain by nurses is often inaccurate, inconsistent or incomplete. For example, in a chart audit of 34 patients with cancer, Paice et al. (1991) found that important aspects of the pain experience (e.g. location, quality, pattern), as well as the effect of analgesics given were inconsistently and poorly documented. Similar findings have been reported by Tittle and McMillan (1994), McMillan and Tittle (1995) and Boegeskov et al. (1994) in an intensive care and post-operative setting, and by O'Connor (1995), Meurier (1998) and Meurier et al.(1998) in a coronary care setting. Furthermore, in an audit following the introduction of a pain assessment chart and care plan into a rehabilitation unit, Carr (1997) found that there was poor linkage between the assessment data and the goals for care and nearly half (44 per cent) of the evaluations did not refer to pain. In a qualitative analysis of nursing documentation of post-operative pain, Briggs and Dean (1998) found that despite the fact that 91 per cent of the patients stated that they experienced pain post-operatively, only 34 per cent of the nurses identified pain as a problem on the care plan. Moreover, it was shown that there was minimal evaluation of the patients' pain experience documented in the care plan.

There are a number of possible reasons for poor documentation of pain. Several researchers have demonstrated that the location of the chart impacts on the quality of pain documentation (Walker and Selmanoff, 1964; Costello and Summers, 1985; Max, 1990; Moody and Snyder, 1995). Meurier et al. (1998) investigated the causes of poor documentation of chest pain assessment by administering a questionnaire to nurses (n=88) working in a general hospital. They found that the most common causes of omissions were the patients' condition, work overload, lack of time, poor assessment documentation, not realising that the assessment had not been fully carried out and different nurses being involved in the assessment of patients. Lack of time, busyness and poor assessment documentation have also been found to be inhibitors of documentation in nursing *per se* (Tapp, 1990; Howse and Bailey, 1992). This gives some indication of the global nature of the problem.

Interpreting Information about Pain

Information about pain must be interpreted in order for either a diagnostic or therapeutic decision to be made (Redmond, in press). This process of interpreting information is thought to be influenced by a number of factors including a nurse's knowledge and experience and the attitudes, values and beliefs he or she holds in relation to pain. Futhermore, large numbers of patient characteristics have been shown to have a significant impact on the nurse's interpretation of information about pain.

Patient characteristics

A nurse's inference of pain is influenced greatly by how a patient expresses pain. Expressive patients are often perceived as being more distressed than stoical patients. This was clearly shown in a study which examined the effect of different levels of non-verbal pain expression on rating of patients' pain (von Baeyer et al., 1984). It was found that nursing students who viewed a short videotape portraying high non-verbal pain expressiveness assigned significantly higher ratings of pain to the patient than those students who viewed a video tape portraying low non-verbal pain expressiveness (von Baeyer et al., 1984). Likewise, in a survey of nurses (n=517) McCaffrey and Ferrell (1994) demonstrated that differences in non-verbal behaviour influenced the respondent's pain assessment in that they were more willing to ascribe pain to the patient who grimaced than the one who smiled, despite the fact that the patients all rated their pain at four on a scale of 0–5. Interestingly, the patients' age made little or no difference to the findings. This has also been shown in a study which employed an experimental 2×2 factorial design to establish the influence of children's vocal expression, age, medical diagnosis and information obtained from parents on paediatric nurses' (n=202) pain assessments (Hamers et al., 1996). The only statistically significant finding was that the subjects attributed more pain to children who expressed their pain vocally than those who did not. However, there was a trend which showed that nurses attributed the most pain to children with a severe diagnosis (defined as closure of anus preaternaturalis).

The patient's diagnosis has been shown to influence nurses' assessment of pain. For example, Dudley and Holm (1984) administered vignettes to randomly selected registered nurses (n=50) and found that the respondents inferred suffering according to the patients' diagnosis. Trauma, in comparison to cardiovascular disease, cancer, infection and psychiatric problems, was viewed as being most physically painful, whereas psychiatric problems were associated with the most psychological distress. Similarly, Taylor et al. (1984) reported that, when presented with descriptions of a hypothetical patient, a sample of American nurses (n=268) were less likely to attribute pain when the patient had no physical pathology present and a pain of long standing duration (low back pain). In a replication of this study, Halfens et al. (1990) found that Dutch nurses (n=133) were also more likely to attribute pain to a hypothetical patient who had significant objective signs of physical pathology, although the nature of the pain (low back, joint or headache) did not influence the nurses' attribution of pain. These differences may have arisen as a result of cultural differences between the two cohorts of nurses or because a sample of qualified nurses was used in one study and a mixture of student and qualified nurses was used in the other.

A number of other researchers have demonstrated that nurses hold negative attitudes towards patients with chronic pain. Teske et al. (1983) compared nurses' observations and patients' self-reports of pain and found that discrepancies between the nurses' and patients' rating of pain were significantly greater with the chronic pain sample. They suggest that this finding is consistent with the belief that patients in chronic pain exaggerate their pain. McKinley and Botti (1991) asked nurses (n=115) to rank the importance of twelve factors they use in deciding a patient's level of pain and found that, for patients with chronic pain, the respondents ranked facial expression as more important than the patient's report of the severity of pain. For other patients they ranked the patient's report of pain severity as more important than facial expression. It would appear that patients with chronic pain are being stereotyped by nurses and this may result in nurses not believing these patients' self-report of pain.

It could be argued that, in general, nurses have difficulty in believing patients' verbal expression of pain. Brockopp et al. (1998) have provided clear evidence to support this assertion in their study on barriers to changes in pain management practice in an acute care setting; they found that nurses were unwilling to believe patients' self-report of pain because of their belief that patients would not accurately report pain levels. Similarly, during in-depth unstructured interviews a group of qualified nurses (n=5) working in surgical units suggested that some patients exaggerate their pain '. . . as an immoral means of securing additional doses of the prescribed medication' (Wakefield, 1995: 906). As a result of this belief they disregarded the patients' pain. Furthermore, Dalton et al. (1998), in a study which examined the impact of an educational programme on nurses' attitudes and pain management practices, reported that prior to the programme 22.8 per cent of the nurses believed that patients' complaints of pain were always real. One year after the programme 81 per cent of them gave this response. Despite this impressive shift in attitude, nearly one-fifth of the nurses still had a problem with believing patients' self-reports of pain.

A number of diverse factors have been shown to influence nurses' assessment of post-operative pain. Zalon (1993) found that the degree of pain experience by post-operative patients influenced nurses' assessment. Nurses (n=119) tended to underestimate severe pain and overestimate mild pain. Moreover, Gujol (1994) administered vignettes to critical care nurses (n=71) and found that the subjects ascribed more pain to the ventilated, as opposed to the non-ventilated, patient despite the fact that in the vignette both patients rated their pain at 4 on a scale of 0–5. In addition, the subjects were more likely to believe the patient's complaints of pain in the early post-operative period. Ventilation status and time since surgery also influenced the nurses' willingness to administer morphine to the patient. Nurses expressed more concern about respiratory depression in non-ventilated patients. It could be argued that these findings indicate that nurses' assessments of post-operative pain are influenced by their misconceptions about the risk of respiratory depression and addiction. They seem to underestimate their patients' pain in order to avoid having to administer a drug about which they harbour considerable concerns.

Nurses' characteristics
Pain assessment is influenced by a number of nurses' characteristics. For example, Davitz et al. (1976) and Davitz and Davitz (1985) have demonstrated that nurses from different cultural backgrounds differ in the degree to which they infer suffering (physical pain and psychological distress) in their patients. Oriental nurses have been found to infer a relatively high level of physical pain, whereas nurses from Western countries tend to infer less pain. This may lead to erroneous clinical decisions whenever nurses care for patients who come from a culture different from their own. For example, nurses who come from a background where dramatic expressions of pain are the norm may underestimate pain intensity in a patient who comes from a culture where stoicism in the face of pain is highly valued.

Mason (1981) used vignettes to examine the factors which influence registered nurses' (n=161) inferences of suffering and found that their years of experience significantly influenced the degree to which they inferred physical pain in patients. Inexperienced nurses tended to infer higher degrees of pain than their more experienced counterparts. Similar findings have been reported by Choiniere et al. (1990) in a study of registered nurses' estimation of pain in patients with severe burn injuries during a therapeutic procedure. In contrast, Halfens et al. (1990) showed that first-year student nurses attributed less pain to a hypothetical patient than third- and fourth-year student nurses and registered nurses. Moreover, Dudley and Holm (1984) demonstrated no significant relationship between years in practice and inference of suffering in a sample of registered nurses. These conflicting findings may have arisen because the samples and methodologies employed in the various studies were quite different.

Again, using the vignette format McCaffrey and Rolling Ferrell (1997) found that when nurses assumed the role of a family member, as opposed to that of the professional nurse, they were more likely to make correct assessments of pain. The authors concluded that when nurses placed themselves in the role of family member, they became more sensitive to the patient's pain. In contrast, when they assumed the role of a nurse they tended to distance themselves from the patient, which reduced their awareness of the patient's needs.

CRITIQUE OF THE METHODS

Over the past two decades a large number of researchers have studied various aspects of the pain assessment process. In general, these studies are poorly reported and subject to a number of methodological weaknesses. Information about the construction, reliability and validity of data collection tools is generally inadequate and most articles do not include a discussion on the limitations of the research. This may reflect the fact that journals have a word count restriction. Unfortunately, the net result is that research consumers will find it difficult to interpret the relevance of the findings and researchers will find many of the studies difficult, if not impossible, to replicate.

In most of the studies, convenience sampling was employed, a weakness further compounded by the fact that in the quantitative studies the sample sizes tended to be very small and response rates were either poorly reported or not identified at all. In a number of surveys the subjects were self selected in that they were attending conferences on pain and it is probable that their responses on pain and its management would be quite different from those of nurses who had never attended a conference on pain. Furthermore, the samples represented a limited number of geographical and healthcare settings and were restricted to a few painful conditions. Sampling in this manner is subject to systematic bias, in that there is a risk that some segment of the population will be systematically under-represented (Polit and Hungler, 1995). It could be argued, therefore, that the findings from these studies should not be generalised to the population as a whole. However, Crombie and Davies (1998) assert that this is not necessarily the case. They state that it is more important to consider how large the bias is and then to assess its potential impact on the conclusions drawn. Unfortunately, because inclusion and exclusion criteria were not identified in many of the studies, and since many of the samples were not well described, it is impossible to undertake such an assessment.

Most of the research designs employed to study aspects of pain assessment are non-experimental and cross-sectional in nature. Such studies have an important role in providing estimates of frequency and in uncovering tentative relationships between variables which can then be tested experimentally. However, sampling bias can have a profound influence on these end-points, and since in most of the studies the degree of bias cannot be determined accurately, caution needs to be exercised when interpreting the results.

A large number of researchers have studied pain assessment using hypothetical clinical situations (vignettes). Vignettes are advantageous in that they are easy to use and take less time than studying real situations. Moreover, they provide strictly controlled conditions which allow different variables to be examined. However, a significant weakness of this data collection approach is that it '. . . tells us what can happen, but not always what does happen in natural settings with many uncontrolled factors' (Carroll and Johnson, 1990: 101). Carroll and Johnson (1990) suggest, therefore, that there is a need for more naturalistic studies, the results from which can then be compared to the hypothetical studies in order to determine which aspects of the decision are the same in both situations.

Decision makers are often unable to articulate how they have made a decision and their memory of a decision situation will fade over time and become mixed up with other memories (Carroll and Johnson, 1990). This has important implications for the study of pain assessment since there is a risk that respondents will not tell the truth because they want to create a favourable impression of themselves or that they may unintentionally reconstruct the decision situation from general know-ledge and any fragments of memory which remain (Carroll and Johnson, 1990). Thus, when nurses are either interviewed about their decisions or asked to answer questions about a hypothetical case, it is possible that they will provide an answer which they think the researcher wants to hear or, alternatively, they will unintentionally distort the decision situation. There may therefore be an inconsistency between what nurses say they do and what they actually do in practice. There is some evidence to show that this is the case with pain assessment (Clarke et al., 1996; Briggs and Dean, 1998). However, this issue has rarely been identified by those who have studied pain assessment, nor has it been addressed as a significant limitation in studies which have employed a survey or interview format.

CONCLUSION

Pain is often an unrelentless and overwhelming experience, the relief of which requires concerted effort on the part of nurses. Assessment is central to successful pain management. This process poses a challenge for nurses, yet there is much evidence to demonstrate that pain assessment practices are sub-optimal and inadequate. This may be because nurses do not appear to give pain assessment a high priority or possibly because pain is essentially a subjective experience which is influenced by a variety of factors, many of which do not seem to be well recognised by nurses. For example, the patient's self report is the single most reliable indicator of pain intensity yet studies indicate that nurses either do not collect data or ignore patients' self reports of pain. Too much emphasis appears to be placed particularly on non-verbal cues in that nurses give priority to what they observe especially when it is inconsistent with the patient's self report. Patients themselves have been shown to be an impediment to optimal pain control since they are often reluctant and sometimes lack the ability to report pain. Pain assessment tools provide patients with a means of overcoming this impediment. Unfortunately, several studies demonstrated that assessment tools are not currently used in clinical practice. Moreover, there is evidence that documentation of pain assessments by nurses is minimal and evaluation is inadequate. Patients' and nurses' characteristics have been found to influence how nurses interpret information about pain. However, the relationship between these factors has not been established conclusively. Indeed, it is by no means clear whether all of the relevant influencing factors have been identified. The factors thought to influence the collection and interpretation of information about pain are summarised in Figure 1. This figure highlights not only the potential negative outcomes of sub-optimal pain assessment for the patient, but also how difficult it would be to establish causal relationships. This review has painted a very negative picture of pain assessment when it is carried out by motivated groups of nurses. If these nurses have not been entirely frank about their practices or have provided a distorted picture of the assessment process, one wonders about the quality of those pain assessments carried out by other, less interested, nurses.

Figure 1. Factors Which Influence Nurses' Assessment of Pain

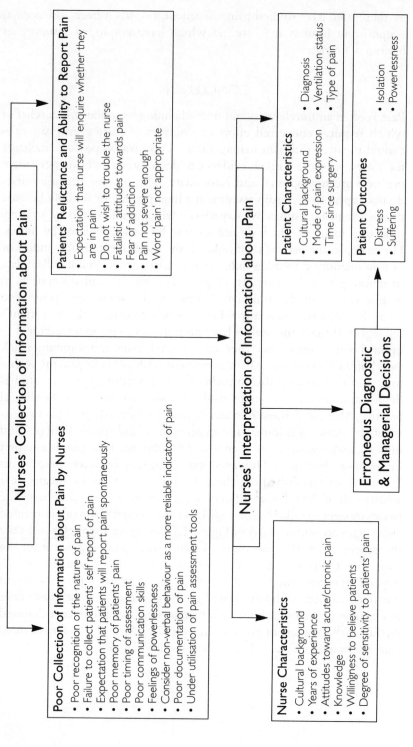

Recommendations for Practice, Education and Future Research

Current pain assessment practices appear to be underpinned by a lack of knowledge about the nature of pain and its treatment and a lack of insight into how the values, attitudes and beliefs held by nurses affect their inferences of pain. Innovative and creative approaches are required to address this situation. Nurses need to be encouraged to collect and interpret information about pain in a more systematic manner and to have their awareness raised about how their values, attitudes and beliefs impact on how they infer pain. One potentially useful approach could be to incorporate some form of pain assessment tool into the flowsheet which is used to document other vital signs. This may help overcome some of the significant barriers to communication which seem to exist in relation to the pain experience, although achieving this end will require intensive effort. Education is probably the single most important means of improving pain assessment practices; however efforts in this area have not proved too successful to date. Nurses need to improve their knowledge about contemporary approaches to the assessment and management of pain. More importantly, however, they need to learn to become more effective in their decision making about pain. This can be achieved by helping them to become aware of the biases that they bring to the decision-making process. They can also be taught to use heuristics such as 'the patient's self-report of pain is the most reliable indicator of pain intensity' in order to avoid these biases and increase their decision-making accuracy. In terms of research, there is a need for more qualitative work in order to provide new insights into and understandings of various dimensions of the pain assessment process. Moreover, there is a need to test whether relationships exist between the many variables identified through non-experimental and qualitative studies. In conclusion, there is a clear need to further our understanding of and develop new approaches to pain assessment. However, achieving improvements in pain assessment is not dependent on such scientific advancement since there is already quite extensive knowledge about this process available. Thus, the greater challenge is to have nurses use available knowledge in an effective and unbiased manner.

REFERENCES

Agency for Health Care Policy and Research (1993) *Acute Pain Management Guidelines*. Rockville, MD: Public Health Service, US Department of Health and Human Services

Agency for Health Care Policy and Research (1994) *Acute Pain Management Guidelines*. Rockville, MD: Public Health Service, US Department of Health and Human Services,

Alleyne, J. and Thomas, V.J. (1994) The management of sickle cell crisis pain as experienced by patients and their carers, *Journal of Advanced Nursing*, 19: 725–32.

Bates, M., Rankin-Hill, L., and Sanchez-Ayendez, M. (1997) The effects of the cultural context of health care on treatment of and response to chronic pain and illness, *Social Science Medicine*, 45: 1433–47.

Bernabei, R., Gambassi, G., Lapane, K., Landi, F., Gatsonis, C., Dunlop, R., Lipsitz, L., Steel, K., and Mor, V. (1998) Management of pain in elderly patients with cancer, *Journal of the American Medical Association*, 23 (279): 1877–82.

Boegeskov Nielsen, L., Svantesson-Martinsson, E., Ingegerd, L., and Bergbom Engberg, L. (1994) An interview study of nurses' assessment and priority of post surgical pain experience, *Intensive and Critical Care Nursing*, 10: 107–14.

Bostrom, B.M., Ramberg, T., Davis, B.D., and Fridlund, B. (1997) Survey of post-operative patient's pain management, *Journal of Nursing Management*, 5: 341–9.

Briggs, M. and Dean, K. (1998) A qualitative analysis of the nursing documentation of post-operative pain management, *Journal of Clinical Nursing*, 7: 155–63.

Brockopp, D., Brockopp, G., Warden, S., Wilson, J., Carpenter, J., and Vandeveer, B. (1998) Barriers to change: a pain management project, *International Journal of Nursing Studies*, 35: 226–32.

Camp, L.D. (1988) A comparison of nurses' recorded assessments of pain with perceptions of pain as described by cancer patients, *Cancer Nursing*, 11: 237–43.

Carr, E. (1990) Postoperative pain: expectations and experiences, *Journal of Advanced Nursing*, 15: 89–100.

Carr, E. (1997) Evaluating the use of a pain assessment tool and care plan: a pilot study. *Journal of Advanced Nursing*, 26: 1073–9.

Carr, E. and Thomas, V.J. (1997) Anticipating and experiencing post-operative pain: the patients' perspective. *Journal of Clinical Nursing*, 6: 191–201.

Carroll, J. and Johnson, E. (1990) *Decision Research*. London: Sage.

Choiniere, M., Melzack, R., Girard, N., Rondeau, J., and Paquin, M.J. (1990) Comparison between patients and nurses assessments of pain and medication efficacy in severe burn injuries, *Pain*, 40: 143–52.

Clarke, E.B., French, B., Bilodeau, M.L., Capasso, V.C., Edwards, A., and Empoliti, J. (1996) Pain management knowledge, attitudes and clinical practice: the impact of nurses' characteristics and education, *Journal of Pain and Symptom Management*, 11 (1): 18–31.

Corner, J. and Wilson–Barnett, J. (1992) The newly registered nurse and the cancer patient: an educational evaluation, *International Journal of Nursing Studies*, 29 (2): 177–90.

Costello, S. and Summers, B. (1985) Documenting patient care: getting it all together, *Nursing Management* 16: 31–4.

Crombie, I.K. and Davies, H.T.O. (1998) Selection bias in pain research, *Pain*, 74: 1–3.

Crow, R.A., Chase, J., and Lamond, D. (1995) The cognitive component of nursing assessment: an analysis, *Journal of Advanced Nursing*, 22: 206–12.

Dalton, J. (1989) Nurses' perceptions of their pain assessment skills, pain management practices, and attitudes toward pain, *Oncology Nursing Forum*, 16: 225–31.

Dalton, J., Carson, J., Mann, J., Blau, W., Bernard, S., and Youngblood, R. (1998) An examination of nursing attitudes and pain management practices, *Cancer Practice*, 6: 115–24.

Davitz, L., Sameshima, Y., and Davitz, J. (1976) Suffering as viewed in six different cultures. *American Journal of Nursing*, 76: 1296–7.

Davitz, L. and Davitz, J. (1985) Culture and nurses' inferences of suffering, in: L.A. Copp (ed.), *Recent Advances in Nursing, Perspectives on Pain*. Edinburgh: Churchill Livingstone: 17–28.

De Schepper, A., Francke, A., and Abu-Saad, H. (1997) Feelings of powerlessness in relation to pain: ascribed causes and reported strategies, *Cancer Nursing*, 20: 422–9.

Dillon McDonald, D. (1996) Nurses' memory of patients' pain, *International Journal of Nursing Studies*, 33: 487–94.

Droogan, J. and Cullum, N. (1998) Systematic reviews in nursing, *International Journal of Nursing Studies*, 35: 13–22.

Dudley, S. and Holm, K. (1984) Assessment of the pain experience in relation to selected nurse characteristics, *Pain*, 18: 179–86.

Eccleston, C., De Williams, A., and Stainton Rogers, W. (1997) Patients and professionals' understandings of the causes of chronic pain: blame, responsibility and identity protection, *Social Science Medicine*, 45: 699–709.

Feldt, K., Warne, M., and Ryden, M. (1998) Examining pain in aggressive cognitively impaired older adults, *Journal of Gerontological Nursing*, November: 14–22.

Ferrell, B., McCaffery, M and Grant, M. (1991) Clinical decision making and pain, *Cancer Nursing*, 14: 289–97.

Ferrell, B., Zichi Cohen, M., Rhiner, M., and Rozek, A. (1991) Pain as a metaphor for illness Part II: family caregivers' management of pain, *Oncology Nursing Forum*, 18: 1315–21.

Field, L. (1996) Factors influencing nurses' analgesia decisions, *British Journal of Nursing*, 5: 838–44.

Fothergill-Bourbonnais, F. and Wilson-Barnett, J. (1992) A comparative study of intensive therapy unit and hospice nurses' knowledge on pain management, *Journal of Advanced Nursing*, 17: 362–72.

Francke, A.L. and Theevven, I. (1994) Inhibition in expressing pain, qualitative study among Dutch surgical breast cancer patients, *Cancer Nursing*, 17: 193–9.

Francke, A., Garssen, B., Huijer Abu-Saad, H., and Grypdonck, M. (1996) Qualitative needs assessment prior to a continuing education program, *Journal of Continuing Education in Nursing*, 27: 34–41.

Gujol, M. (1994) A survey of pain assessment and management practices among critical care nurses, *American Journal of Critical Care*, 3: 123–8.

Hadjistavropoulos, H.D., Craig, K., Hadjistavropoulos, T., and Poole, G. (1996) Subjective judgements of deceptions in pain expression: accuracy and errors, *Pain*, 65: 251–8.

Halfens, R., Evers, G., and Abu-Saad, H. (1990) Determinants of pain assessment by nurses, *International Journal of Nursing Studies*, 27: 43–9.

Hamers, J.P.H., Abu-Saad, H.H., van den Hout, M.A., Halfens, R.J.G., and Kester, A.D.M. (1996) The influence of children's vocal expression, age, medical diagnosis and information obtained from parents on nurses' pain assessments and decisions regarding interventions, *Pain*, 65: 53–61.

Harrison, A. (1991) Assessing patients' pain: identifying reasons for error, *Journal of Advanced Nursing*, 16: 1018–25.

Harrison, A., Ahmed Busabir, A., Obeid AL-Kaabi, A., and Khalid AL-Awadi, H. (1996) Does sharing a mother-tongue affect how closely patients and nurses agree when rating the patient's pain, worry and knowledge? *Journal of Advanced Nursing*, 24: 229–35.

Hartford, M., Karlson, B., Sjolin, M., Holmberg, S., and Herlitz, J. (1993) Symptoms, thoughts, and environmental factors in suspected acute myocardial infarction, *Heart and Lung*, 22: 64–70.

Hawthorn, J. and Redmond, K. (1998) *Pain: Causes and Management.* Oxford: Blackwell.

Hofgren, C., Karlson, B., Gaston-Johansson, F., and Herlitz, J. (1994) Word descriptors in suspected acute myocardial infarction: a comparison between patients with and without combined myocardial infarction, *Heart and Lung*, 23: 397–403.

Howse, E. and Bailey, J. (1992) Resistance to documentation – a nursing research issue, *International Journal of Nursing Studies*, 29 (4): 371–80.

Juhl, I., Christensen, B., Bulow, H., Wilbek, H., Dreifer, W., and Egelund, B. (1993) Post operative pain relief from the patients' and nurses' point of view, *Acta Anaesthesiologica Scandinavica*, 37: 404–9.

Lamond, D., Crow, R., Chase, J., Doggen, K., and Swinkels, M. (1996) Information sources used in decision making: considerations for simulation development, *International Journal of Nursing Studies*, 33 (1): 47–57.

Lenz, E.R., Pugh, L.C., Milligan, R.A., Gift, A., and Suppe, F. (1997) The middle-range theory of unpleasant symptoms: An update, *Advances in Nursing Science* 19 (3): 14–27.

McCaffrey, M. and Ferrell, B. (1991) How would you respond to these patients in pain? *Nursing 91*, 21: 34–7.

McCaffrey, M. and Ferrell, B. (1994) Nurses' assessment of pain intensity and choice of analgesic dose, *Contemporary Nurse*, 3: 68–74.

McCaffrey, M. and Rolling Ferrell, B. (1997) Influence of professional role on pain assessment and use of opioids, *Journal of Continuing Education in Nursing*, 28: 69–77.

McKinley, and Botti, M. (1991) Nurses' assessment of pain in hospitalised patients, *The Australian Journal of Advanced Nursing*, 9: 7–14.

Mackintosh, C. (1994) Non-reporting of cardiac pain: why do patients in a CCU fail to report pain, *Nursing Times* 90: 36–9.

McMillan, S.C. and Tittle, M. (1995) A descriptive study of management of pain and pain related side effects in a cancer centre and a hospice, *Hospice Journal* 10: 89–107.

Mason, D. (1981) An investigation of the influences of selected factors on nurses inferences of patient suffering, *International Journal of Nursing Studies*, 18: 251–9.

Max, M.B. (1990) Improving outcomes of analgesic treatment: is education enough? *Annals of Internal Medicine*, 113: 885–9.

Meehan, D., McRae, M.E., Rourke, D.A., Eisenring, C., and Imperial, F.A. (1995) Analgesic administration, pain intensity and patient satisfaction in cardiac surgical patients, *American Journal of Critical Care* 4: 435–42.

Meurier, C.E. (1998) The quality of assessment of patients with chest pain: the development of a questionnaire to audit the nursing assessment record of patients with chest pain, *Journal of Advanced Nursing*, 27: 140–6.

Meurier, C.E., Vincent, C.A., and Parmar, D.G. (1998) Perception of causes of omissions in the assessment of patients with chest pain, *Journal of Advanced Nursing*, 28: 1012–19.

Moody, L. and Synder, P.E. (1995) Hospital provider satisfaction with a new documentation system, *Nursing Economics* 13: 24–31.

Nagy, S. (1998) A comparison of the effects of patients' pain on nurses working in burns and neonatal care units, *Journal of Advanced Nursing*, 27: 335–40

Nash, R., Edwards, H., and Nebauer, M. (1993) Effects of attitudes, subjective norms and perceived control on nurses' intention to assess patients' pain, *Journal of Advanced Nursing*, 18: 941–7.

O' Connor, L. (1995) Pain assessments by patients and nurses and nurses notes on it in early acute myocardial infarction. Part II. *Intensive and Critical Care Nursing*, 11: 283–92.

O'Brien, S., Dalton, J., Konsler, G., and Carlson, J. (1996) The knowledge and attitudes of experienced oncology nurses regarding the management of cancer-related pain, *Oncology Nursing Forum*, 23 (3): 515–22.

Paice, J., Mahon, S., and Faut-Callahan, M. (1991) Factors associated with adequate pain control in hospitalised postsurgical patients diagnosed with cancer, *Cancer Nursing*, 14: 298–305.

Polit, D.E., and Hungler, B. (1995) *Nursing Research: Principles and Methods,* Philadelphia: J.B. Lippincott.

Redmond, K. (1998) Barriers to the effective management of pain, *International Journal of Palliative Nursing*, 4 (6): 276–83

Redmond, K. (in press) Clinical decision making, in: N Kearney and A. Richardson (eds), *Advanced Practice in Cancer Nursing*. Edinburgh: Churchill Livingstone.

Renfroe, D., O'Sullivan, P., and McGee, G. (1990) The relationship of attitude, subjective norm and behavioural intent to the documentation behaviour of nurses, *Scholarly Inquiry for Nursing Practice*, 4: 47–60.

Riddell, A. and Fitch, M.I. (1997) Patients' knowledge and attitudes towards the management of cancer pain, *Oncology Nursing Forum*, 24 (10): 1775–88.

Scheider, A. (1987) Unreported chest pain in a coronary care unit, *Focus on Critical Care,* 14: 21–4.

Schwartz, J. and Keller, C. (1993) Variables affecting the reporting of pain following an acute myocardial infarction, *Applied Nursing Research*, 6: 13–18.

Scott, L.E. (1992) Effectiveness of documented assessment of postoperative pain, *British Journal of Nursing*, 3: 494–501.

Seers, K. (1987) 'Peceptions of pain, *Nursing Times*, 83, 37–9.

Stephenson, N. L. (1994) A comparison of nurse and patient, *Journal of Intravenous Nursing*, 17: 235–9.

Sun, X. and Weissman, C. (1994) The use of analgesics and sedatives in critically ill patients: physicians' orders versus medications administered, *Heart and Lung* 23: 169–76.

Sutters, K.A. and Miaskowski, C. (1992) The problem of pain in children with cancer: a research review, *Oncology Nursing Forum* 19: 465–71.

Tapp, R.A. (1990) Inhibitors and facilitators to documentation of nursing practice, *Western Journal of Nursing Research*, 12 (2): 229–40.

Taylor, A.G., Skelton, J., and Butcher, J. (1984) Duration of pain condition and physical pathology as determinants of nurses' assessments of patients in pain, *Nursing Research*, 33: 4–8.

Teske, K., Daut, R.L., and Cleeland, C.S. (1983) Relationships between nurses' observations and patients' self-reports of pain, *Pain*, 16: 289–96.

Tittle, M. and McMillan, S.C. (1994) Pain and pain related side effects in a ICU and on a surgical unit nurses' management, *American Journal of Critical Care*, 3: 25–30.

von Baeyer, C.L., Johnson, M.E., and McMillan, M.J. (1984) Consequences of non verbal expression of pain: patient distress and observer concern, *Social Science and Medicine*, 19: 1319–24.

Vortherms, R., Ryan, P., and Ward, S. (1992) Knowledge of, attitudes toward, and barriers to pharmacologic management of cancer pain in a statewide random sample of nurses, *Research in Nursing and Health*, 15: 459–66.

Waddie, N.A. (1996) Language and pain expression, *Journal of Advanced Nursing*, 23: 868–72.

Wakefield, A. (1995) Pain: an account of nurses' talk, *Journal of Advanced Nursing*, 21: 905–10.

Walker, J.H., Akinsanya, J.A., Davis, B.D., and Marcer, D. (1990) The nursing management of elderly patients with pain in the community: study and recommendations, *Journal of Advanced Nursing*, 15: 1154–61.

Walker, V.H., and Selmanoff, E.D. (1964) A study of the nature and uses of nurses' notes, *Nursing Research*, 13: 113–21.

Wilkie, D.J., Williams, A.R., Grevstad, P., and Mekwa, J. (1995) Coaching persons with lung cancer to report sensory pain, *Cancer Nursing*, 18: 7–15.

Wilkinson, S. (1991) Factors which influence how nurses communicate with cancer patients, *Journal of Advanced Nursing*, 16: 677–88.

Willetts, K. (1989) Assessing cardiac pain, *Nursing Times*, 85: 52–4.

Winefield, H., Katsikitis, M., Hart, L.M., and Rounsefell, B.F. (1990) Postoperative pain experiences: relevant patient and staff attitudes, *Journal of Psychosomatic Research*, 34: 543–52.

World Health Organisation (WHO) (1996) *Cancer Pain Relief. WHO Technical Report Series*. Geneva: WHO.

Yates, P., Dewar, A., and Fentiman, B. (1995) Pain: the views of elderly people living in long-term residential care settings, *Journal of Advanced Nursing*, 21: 667–74.

Zalon, M. (1993) Nurses' assessment of postoperative patients' pain, *Pain*, 54: 329–34.

Zalon, M. (1997) Pain in frail elderly women after surgery, *Image: Journal of Nursing Scholarly Inquiry*, 29: 21–6.

9

Patients' Experiences of In-Patient Mental Health Care

Mary Farrelly

INTRODUCTION AND BACKGROUND TO THE STUDY

This study explores patients' experiences of acute in-patient mental health care using a phenomenological approach. The increasing level of consumerism in society is placing an imperative on service providers to consider the views of users of services in service evaluation and planning. The mentally ill is a group that has traditionally been marginalised within society and although there is a growing recognition of the rights of the mentally ill to self determination and involvement in care, this right to involvement is still not universally accepted.

Sines (1994: 901) has suggested that :

> the challenge for mental health nurses must be to reverse the process by which professional intent is perceived as being arrogant.

Listening to what patients have to say is one way of doing this. Patients' opinions of mental health care have mostly been sought in the context of patient satisfaction surveys. While valuable information has been gained from such surveys, they are limited in the information that they elicit by the constraints of the methods adopted. There is scope for new ways to be found for patients to tell their stories. This study aims to tell patients' stories in a way that is true to their experiences and meaningful to those providing services for them and a phenomenological approach has been adopted to achieve this.

In the quantitive paradigm, data are collected using instruments that are constructed by the researchers, which may reflect the priorities and concerns of the professionals and managers rather than the patients. The majority of studies on the topic under consideration here have been small scale and have provided scant information about methodological procedures, thus making generalisations difficult. Quantitative approaches limit the depth of information that can be elicited, restricting the individual to responses that can be measured. Results achieved using these methods have been mixed, with both positive and negative opinions expressed. There are, however, many methodological difficulties inherent in measuring a subjective concept such as satisfaction; how, when, where and by whom instruments are administered may affect the results achieved. When qualitative approaches are adopted, the results tend to be more critical and reasons for dissatisfaction are explained and clarified. There are few studies that have explored patients' experiences of mental health care in any in-depth way, allowing their priorities to emerge, and no such studies have been carried out in Ireland.

RESEARCH DESIGN

The research question asked in this study was: how does a person experience being a patient in an acute psychiatric ward? A phenomenological approach was adopted. Phenomenology is concerned with the lived experience of people; its central aim is tell their true story in the way that they would tell it themselves.

Phenomenology began as a philosophy and also developed as an approach to the study of the human experience. When applied as a research approach it fits within the qualitative paradigm. The term phenomenology stems from the Greek word 'phainein', which means to show, to be seen or to appear (Holloway and Wheeler, 1996). Phenomenology is most commonly described as the study of lived experience (Van Manen, 1984; Holloway and Wheeler, 1996). Spiegelberg (1975: 3, cited by Streubert and Carpenter, 1995) defines it as:

> the name for a philosophical movement whose primary objective is the direct investigation and description of phenomena as consciously experienced, without theories about their causal explanation and as free as possible from unexamined preconceptions and presuppositions.

It endeavours to arrive at the true meaning of an experience for an individual or group as it is immediately experienced rather than how it is conceptualised or categorised by them (Van Manen, 1984).

Several concepts are fundamental to phenomenology. These are essences, intuiting and phenomenological reduction. Essences refer to the elements related to the true meaning of something or the basic units of common understanding (Streubert and Carpenter, 1995). Intuiting is the process of accurate interpretation of the data so that a common understanding is reached (Streubert and Carpenter, 1995) and involves the researcher focusing all awareness and energy on the data in order to increase insight (Burns and Grove, 1987). Phenomenological reduction refers to 'epoche' in the words of Husserl, which literally means suspension of belief (Holloway and Wheeler, 1996). Van Manen (1984) has noted that the problem in phenomenological inquiry is not always that we know too little about a phenomenon but that we know too much. Phenomenological reduction refers to an attempt to address this in that it requires the researcher first to identify any preconceived notions or ideas about the phenomenon under investigation and to use a technique of 'bracketing' out prior assumptions, beliefs, preconceptions and biases in order to experience the phenomenon naively (Streubert and Carpenter, 1995; Morse, 1991). Merleau-Ponty (1956, cited by Streubert and Carpenter, 1995) has commented that this may not be completely possible because of the intimate nature of the relationship that people have with the world. It is suggested, however, that what can be achieved is to make explicit our understandings, beliefs, biases, assumptions and presumptions so that we are aware of them and attempt to forget them as we approach the data (Van Manen, 1984).

The aim of this study is to explore the experiences of patients who have been in acute psychiatric wards. The commitment within phenomenology to the participant's personal experience makes it a suitable approach to fulfil the aim of this study.

DATA COLLECTION

Negotiating Access to the Research Site

Permission was sought in writing of the hospital ethics committee and all members were furnished with a copy of the research proposal. The researcher attended a committee meeting in order to respond to any queries that the committee had in relation to the proposal. The permission of the ethics committee was withheld pending legal advice on a number of aspects of the research design. These were in relation to providing the researcher with discharge records in order to access the sample and exclude psychotic patients. Legal opinion concurred with the proposal of the researcher and so permission was granted.

The next level of negotiation of access was with the potential participants. When the sample was selected, the researcher contacted all potential participants by phone. She introduced herself and explained the nature of the study and what would be required of them if they chose to participate. This included information about audiotaping the interviews. They were assured of the voluntary nature of participation and issues of confidentiality and anonymity were guaranteed. If they initially indicated a negative response the researcher terminated the conversation expressing thanks for their time. Those who expressed interest were then offered a choice of location, and a mutually suitable time and place were agreed. Participants were given the researcher's phone number if they needed to establish contact to change or cancel the arrangements.

Sample Selection

Initially it had been decided that a purposeful sample would be selected using six selection criteria. These were that they would be patients who:

1 had a first admission to a psychiatric ward within the previous six months in order to facilitate accurate recall;

2 had been discharged over one month previously in order to maximise the chances that they would feel free from the hospital setting and feel able to be open and honest about their experiences;

3 were over 18 years of age to eliminate the necessity for parental consent;

4 had received care in a public psychiatric ward as it was assumed that there would be differences in the experiences of those who had received care in private facilities;

5 were in hospital on a voluntary basis;

6 were not currently psychotic. This was not to minimise their experiences in any way but to limit the amount of distress that might be caused through the reliving of their experiences and ensure that accounts of hospitalisation were not influenced by current symptomatology;

7 had not been under the care of the researcher at any time in order to maximise the chances of them feeling free to express themselves honestly and openly.

Discharge records were examined and attempts were made to contact those people who fulfilled the criteria. It was not possible to identify those who were psychotic from these records and so it was decided that this judgement would be made by the researcher, either at initial contact or in the interview setting. A sufficient number of participants were not sourced following these procedures. This occurred for several reasons. Firstly, only a small number of those discharged in the past six months were first time admissions. A number of these had changed address and were not contactable. Of those that were contactable a number refused to participate. Although frustrating from a research perspective, this was viewed positively by the researcher, since it was clear that the methods employed to recruit people for the research were not viewed by the participants as coercive and that they did not feel compelled to participate. Owing to these difficulties in recruiting the sample it was not possible to adhere to the original selection criteria.

As an adequate sample could not be selected using the selection criteria, it was necessary to alter the sampling strategy. A wider group was contacted in order to achieve sufficient numbers. Nurses working in day services (i.e. day hospitals, day centres, out-patient clinics and substance abuse services) were informed of the nature of the research and were requested to ask their clients if they would be interested in participating. This constituted a process of volunteer sampling (Morse, 1991). The technique was successful in eliciting a sufficient number of participants, although it is acknowledged it may have adversely affected the study. Firstly as the researcher had no control over who was asked, the nurses may have exercised discretion in those they asked to participate – for example they may have consciously or unconsciously selected patients likely to give favourable responses. Secondly, the experiences of a volunteer sample may differ from that elicited otherwise in that they may hold very definite views (either positive or negative).

Description of the Sample

In all 13 people were contacted and eight agreed to take part. All of the participants had received care in public psychiatric wards. The researcher had not been involved in caring for the participants at any time. The average age of the participants was 41 years, with a range from 23 to 57 years. Three of the participants were male and five were female.

Collection of Data

Data collection took place over a period of three weeks and consisted of eight audio-taped interviews. A pilot interview was carried out to familiarise the researcher with the interview process and to identify any difficulties that might arise in the study. This pilot interview was transcribed and examined by the researcher to evaluate the quality of the interview technique. The importance of assisting the participant to focus on the topic was noted during the interview as the participant tended to go on to discuss other issues. This had to be balanced with a sensitivity to the participant's feelings. The researcher became aware of the need to make a judgement about when to allow a person to continue to talk about personal issues that might not be of particular relevance to the aim of the research or when to attempt to focus him or her, since the participant should always take precedence over the aims of the research. It was decided that this pilot interview yielded sufficient information to warrant its inclusion in the study.

Four of the interviews took place in the participants' homes and four took place in the care centre that they attended. All of the settings were chosen by the participants. The interviews lasted between half an hour and ninety minutes. The interviews began with a clarification of the purpose of the research, a statement about issues of confidentiality and anonymity, a reassurance to the participant that he or she could terminate the interview or withdraw consent at any stage if he or she so wished, and a reminder about the use of the tape recorder. They were then asked to sign a consent form restating these issues.

The interviews then progressed with the researcher asking participants to describe what it was like for them to be admitted to a psychiatric hospital. If necessary, probing questions were asked. At the end of the interview if participants had expressed mainly positive views they were asked if they had had any negative experiences to recount and vice versa. They were also asked if there was anything else that they felt they wanted to add or if there was anything that the researcher had omitted (Morse and Field, 1995). If the participants had difficulty in elaborating on their experiences then they were asked about different aspects of care as identified in previous interviews with other participants and in themes already generated in the literature.

'Bracketing' was attempted as far as was possible by the researcher and to facilitate this process some time was taken prior to each interview to reflect on the researcher's thoughts and feelings on entering the research site, and to rehearse the questions and initial interaction with the participant. Every attempt was made in the course of the interviews not to guide the participant in any particular way.

Data Analysis

Data analysis was carried out in accordance with the guidelines outlined in Streubert's ten step process as outlined below.

1   The researcher explicates a personal description of the phenomenon of interest.

2   The researcher examines his/her presuppositions and preconceived ideas about the phenomenon and attempts to 'bracket' them.

3   The participants are interviewed in unfamiliar settings.

4   All of the transcripts are read by the researcher in order to obtain a general sense of the experience that the participants have described.

5   The transcripts are reviewed to uncover essences. Essences are common themes that emerge in the data.

6   Patterns of essential relationships are established.

7   Formalised descriptions of the phenomena are then developed.

8 The researcher returns to the participants to validate the descriptions that have been formulated.

9 The relevant literature is reviewed.

10 The findings of the study are disseminated to the nursing community.

(Streubert, 1991)

All of the interviews were transcribed in type. Two copies were made: a master copy for safe keeping and a second copy for thematic analysis. All of the transcripts were read several times so that the researcher would become familiar with the content. All key phrases and statements that pertained to the research question were extracted and stored separately. Each of these statements or phrases was examined to uncover essences. The data were then re-read to explicate essential relationships and through this process themes were established. Description of these themes was then carried out and compared back to the original data to ensure that the issues that were stated by the participants were accurately represented. Although this is shown here as a linear process, the researcher in fact found that the process of data analysis began soon after completion of the first interview and continued during the data collection phase. Meanings and themes began to emerge in the researcher's mind during this time, which were either retained or rejected, on the basis of further data collection and formal data analysis. The researcher recognised that it was necessary to engage in 'bracketing' to deal with this process, as it was important to recognise the danger that themes could have been formulated at too early a stage in the research process which, if not recognised, could have led to premature closure and superficial or incomplete data collection and analysis.

Issues of Rigour

Two processes were carried out in order to enhance the credibility of this study. First, a copy of the themes that were generated from the data was given to two of the participants of the study. They were asked to read through them and to comment on whether they felt that they accurately represented their experiences. Both participants confirmed that the themes generated accurately represented their experiences.

Secondly, two independent experts (experienced psychiatric nurses) were given a copy of the findings together with copies of the transcripts and they were asked to compare the researcher's thematic analysis with their own. No differences were found in the generation of themes. On discussion with the academic supervisor it was decided to change the title of one theme, which it was felt did not accurately represent all of the data contained in it and to further subdivide another theme to facilitate clearer understanding of the data.

FINDINGS

Six themes emerged from the analysis of the data on the experiences of the participants of acute in-patient psychiatric care. They were:

• encounters with other patients
• pharmacological and non-pharmacological therapies
• loss of control and freedom
• staff attitudes
• someone to talk to
• physical amenities

Details of the essences that were uncovered in the formulation of these themes are provided in Table 1.

Encounters with Other Patients

Other patients featured largely in the participants' experiences of being in hospital. Experiences with other patients were a constant and pervasive source of fear for the participants in this study. The fact that patients with a variety of different illnesses and of differing levels of severity were treated in the same wards was commented on. The participants found the bizarre behaviour of other patients disturbing. For example as Informant 01 says:

> Well there'd be patients sitting there and they'd be talking to themselves, screaming, and like that's very frightening. Like you're just sitting there and you don't know what's going to happen next and then if they start getting bad like the panic button goes and you're thrown out of the room and you just hear the patient screaming and getting the injection.

This would occur in the common areas of the wards when they encountered other patients, such as in the smoking or sitting rooms, as Informant 02 says:

> And then the smoking room like I mean, I used to go into regularly. That was just terrible experience. It really freaked me. You know people would just start staring at you, and you know and then if you looked at them, what are you looking at, you know. And like you just wanted a smoke, you know. So that place freaked me out . . . But I really, really felt intimidated now. I felt I was going to be killed there. This girl she was terrifying, 'cos she was a huge big girl like, if she wanted to make mincemeat of you she would. But there was another few like just sit there

Table 1. Essences and Themes Uncovered in Data Analysis.

Essences	Themes
Other patients' disruptive behaviour	ENCOUNTERS WITH OTHER PATIENTS
Fear	
Meeting someone you know	
Physical assaults	
Verbal assaults	
Gender mix	
Property stolen	
Forming friendships	
Medication	PHARMACOLOGICAL AND NON-
Side effects	PHARMACOLOGICAL THERAPIES
Group therapy	
Relaxation	
Helpfulness	
Choice	
Passing the time	
Being locked up	LOSS OF CONTROL AND FREEDOM
Not involved in decisions	
Compelled to comply with therapies	
Lack of information	
Flexibility	STAFF ATTITUDES
Kindness	
Uncaring	
Talking	SOMEONE TO TALK TO
Listening	
Primary nurses	
No time	
Food	PHYSICAL AMENITIES
Geography of ward	
Bedrooms	
Décor	
Effect on mood	

and they would just from the medication, I don't know what. But they'd just start looking at you and I'd feel very uncomfortable like. They really would stare you like, you'd be sort of terrified, like you know.

The participants did not mention these feelings to the staff as they perceived the staff to be too busy to deal with issues that might be viewed as trivial.

> MF: But you didn't feel able to talk to anyone about that?
> Informant 02: No I didn't actually you know.

One participant reported that some of her property was stolen and items of clothing burnt with cigarettes while she was in hospital. Another reported two assaults on her, one in which a male visitor of another patient started to kiss her and another in which another patient without provocation headbutted her. Neither of these incidents was witnessed by or reported to staff. She went on to describe her perception of the environment:

> Informant 03: It's a hard environment, like going to prison only the tough survive it like . . .

and the lasting effect that the experience had on her:

> Informant 03: When I was leaving I was, the only difference between when I was admitted and when I was leaving was the elation was gone. But I was still the same person the whole time so by the time I was leaving, the hospital had made its mark on me all the experiences that I'd been through and I left with that mark, when I left like you don't just suddenly wake up, you're the same person when you're manic as when you're well. Same intelligence, same thoughts. So when I left the hospital it was just a joy to leave.

The practice that is now common in many general and psychiatric hospitals of having men and women cared for in the same wards was criticised by some of the female participants. They commented on the state of dress of some male patients who were unwell and the sometimes uninhibited behaviour in which they engaged, which they found disturbing and threatening. One participant met a neighbour while in hospital and commented that this made him feel uncomfortable as he felt she would tell other people that he was in a psychiatric ward.

While some of the participants reported that they found it helpful to talk to some of the other patients who were not so disturbed, and had indeed made friends among them, these experiences were not explored by them in as great a depth as the negative experiences that they had.

Pharmacological and Non-Pharmacological Therapies

This theme relates to therapies that the participants experienced while in hospital. The therapies fell into two distinct categories – pharmacological and non-pharmacological therapies – which will be discussed separately.

Pharmacological therapies

Medication was felt to be a large part of the treatment that they received. All the participants received some medication and while some felt that it was helpful, others found it to be of no use. Some side effects were experienced by the participants, most commonly drowsiness, restlessness and in one case nausea and vomiting. One participant felt that medication was given too much when what was required was just an opportunity to talk. In Informant 01's own words:

> Because, all the people, well it's not all they really need, but most of the time, you just need someone to talk to, to try and help them sort out what's going on in their head. That's all they need, instead of the medication. I know people need medication but not half of the stuff they're on, doped up and that.

Another participant described the trauma of being detoxified from alcohol and librium:

> Informant 04: Yeah that was awful, the worst experience I've ever had in me life, only I had a strong heart, I'd say I'd be dead. I mean that cos I was shaking, it was like as if someone took a string out of my stomach say, like a violin string, and just pulled it out like that a couple of feet and then it go ping.

This he felt had occurred too quickly and without his consent.

Non-pharmacological therapies

Non-pharmacological therapies mentioned by the participants were primarily group activities that the participants experienced and included arts and crafts, bingo, relaxation, stress awareness groups and physical exercises. Relaxation was mentioned repeatedly as being a most enjoyable and helpful form of therapy. It was described in glowing terms which indicated the extent of its perceived value to the participants. As Informant 03 said:

> . . . there was one that was like wonderful and that was relaxation therapy. They turned one of the rooms, a beautifully carpeted room, you'd lie down on the floor and there was a big bubble machine. And it worked on all the patients and the patients loved it. It was the one thing that everyone wanted to, the only thing that people like to do. And you go into the room and you lie on the floor and you'd relax.

Other group therapeutic activities were experienced in different ways by the participants. Some found them useful, while others felt that they were of no value. Common to all the participants, however, was the view that the principal value of the planned group activities provided in the wards was that they helped to pass the time.

> Informant 02: . . . except maybe that activities are really important 'cos the days are really long . . . You just sort of sit there and you're concentrating. Instead of lying and thinking about yourself, when am I ever going to get out of here. You completely forget about that and [nurse's name] would put on the music and there would be a bit of chit chat and a bit of slagging going on and you know. It'd be friendly like you know. So it'd be grand and it'd be hours so your whole afternoon would be gone.

There appeared to be no matching of patients to therapeutic activities suitable to their particular needs. Some stated that they were unable to take part in certain activities owing to aspects of their illness or other personal reasons. All the participants felt that they were compelled to attend general group activities by the staff. This will be explored in more depth in the section relating to personal choice.

Loss of Control and Freedom

Many of the participants' reported feeling that they had lost control over their lives while in hospital was coupled with experiencing loss of personal freedom in the wards. This referred both to the lack of physical freedom of not being able to leave the ward when they wished and of not being involved in decisions made about their own care. It was acknowledged by some that owing to the acuity of their illness in the early stages they might not have been able to participate meaningfully in decisions about their care but that this was not the case for the full length of their stay. They felt that they would have welcomed more opportunities to become involved and be consulted about their condition and their care. For example:

> MF: While you were there did you feel that you were able to participate in decisions about your care or about what was happening to you?
> Informant 02: No, not really that was all kind of decided and planned out really, I thought. By the staff really . . .
> MF: Did you feel that you would have liked to be more involved or you would have been able to be more involved?
> Informant 02: Ahm yeah well you have your own ideas really like I mean you know yourself best really don't you so it wouldn't do any harm. Probably not in the first few days when you're admitted, 'cos you're probably a bit stupid anyway you know but when you're a little bit

well, more well maybe it's then at that stage that you know what you think you know. Just a few thoughts probably wouldn't go amiss really . . . it would be nice to have more of a say in your own development and your own kind of recovery kind of. 'Cos you know yourself best and you can give the reasons why you're thinking a certain way and you can argue a point as such you know and then even if you don't succeed like at least you put your own view forward.

All the participants reported being in locked environments which they could not leave without permission. This included those who were in hospital as voluntary patients as well as those who were of involuntary (or temporary[1]) status. In Informant 05's words:

MF: What other things stick in your mind about being in hospital then?
Informant 05: Well being enclosed really. The door's locked you know what I mean. And you had no freedom.
MF: And how did that make you feel?
Informant 05: It made me feel sad really, in a way you know.
MF: Why?
Informant 05: Well that you lost your freedom in the first place, you know.
MF: Were the doors closed all the time?
Informant 05: Well not all the time, when the visiting hours were on the doors were open but I didn't never went outside like you know I stayed in. Then when you when the bell went or at time for people to go you could hear the doors being closed and you knew that you're kind of locked in again.

Both groups, those who were voluntary and temporary, had their day clothes taken from them by staff and were compelled to spend the days in nightclothes.

MF: How did you feel about going into hospital, into a psychiatric ward?
Informant 06: Brutal, the worst thing that ever happened me. I thought that I was mad. I wasn't mad. I knew I wasn't mad. I just couldn't help myself. Then the nurse came along and he took my clothes and I thought I'm locked up, I must be mad if they take me clothes and that.

Participants felt compelled to comply with treatment regimens, both medication and group therapeutic activities. They experienced pressure from staff to attend group activities whether they wanted to or not, even to the extent that other areas of the ward were being locked so that they would have no option but to attend. For example in Informant 06's words:

[The nurse said . . .] you have to go up to the activities. I said, 'What?' So I didn't know where the activities were or anything. He says we're locking the wards at 10.30. I said you're locking the wards at 10.30, why? He said we just do that you know . . . So at 10.30 the ward was locked, not being able to walk down the corridor. You had to take part in this, and you had to do this and you had to that. In the [name of other hospital] if you didn't want to do it you didn't have to do it. Someone would come and talk to you like you know what I mean?

Staff Attitudes

Staff mentioned by the participants were primarily nursing and medical staff. Both groups were experienced as individuals rather than as distinct groups by the various participants in the study. Some staff were perceived to be kind and helpful, while others were perceived not to care or understand participants' particular problems. One participant describes how a nurse helped him out of an awkward situation:

> Informant 06: And me brother was home from America well, he was due home from America and I told the nurses that I didn't want to see him. So fair play he did come in and the nurse came over and said, 'You have to go down for therapy now, you know', so that got rid of him.

Flexibility within the ward environment and routine was highly valued and this appeared to be linked by the participants to the attitudes and behaviour of the nursing staff. Informant 06 described being unable to sleep and compared two different approaches that he experienced:

> But there was one night there I asked for a cup of tea I couldn't sleep and I was just sitting there at the side of the bed. There was nothing to do and there was nowhere to go and the nurse comes in, she was real abrupt said there's no tea here after such and such an hour and that's it. And I said f__ you to meself, so I just lay there on the bed but I didn't sleep. And they knew I wasn't sleep, they were coming in checking you know. In [name of other hospital] at least they'd come in and if you were not sleeping they'd say are you all right you know, do you want to talk or something. And I could hear them having their supper laughing and talking outside.

The participants were able to identify different approaches that staff took to patients and valued staff who demonstrated kindness, understanding and caring. They criticised staff whom they perceived to be domineering or uncaring.

> Informant 06: When you were in [name of hospital] if you were smoking like in the dining room they'd come and tell you not to smoke even the real heavy smokers. And they wouldn't get annoyed at you, they'd just get up and go to the smokers' room. It was just a different way of doing it. I mean they just had a different approach. It wasn't a domineering approach. In [name of other hospital] it was a domineering approach, you had to do this and you had to do that.

While all staff were perceived as being busy and not as available as often as the participants would like, some staff who were helpful to them were remembered and appreciated. For example:

> MF: What would you say was what kind of things were helpful?
> Informant 05: Aah well the staff were kind and they looked after me you know.

And

> Informant 02: The first time I was a bit scared really, 'cos it was so big like and I was used to the smallness of [name of private ward]. But they were very good, eh the psychiatric nurses, introduced me like, brought me off and explained everything to me. You know very reassuring.

Doctors were similarly mentioned:

> Informant 03: And then I found like when I was in there, [name of doctor] was my doctor. And she was brilliant like, she was just, she got me so much better.

Someone to Talk to

Having someone to talk to emerged as being important to participants in their experiences of being in psychiatric wards. They felt that being able to talk to someone, a nurse or a doctor who had time to listen, helped in their recovery. For example:

> Informant 06: Then the nurse came in a sat beside me and we talked. It relieved me a little bit, he has the patience to listen, you know. It helped that someone was able to listen not running off, you know.

It was particularly mentioned by them when staff sought them out to discuss their problems. In areas that organised nursing care on a primary nursing or key worker system this was noted by the participants. The role of the primary nurse in listening and talking was valued by the patients:

> Informant 06: Em, you had, each senior nurse had a certain amount of people to look after, you probably know about that. But they'd come and they'd talk to you or they'd call you into the room and they'd talk to you and they'd stay there until you were finished talking you know they wouldn't be rushing out.

but it was also noted if the primary nurse failed to fulfil this role:

> MF: Did you know who your key nurse was?
> Informant 01: Yeah when I first went in she says, 'I'm your key nurse' but that was it.
> MF: So you didn't see her after that?
> Informant 01: No, well only when I was going.

Positive experiences were mentioned where the participants found staff available and willing to listen and discuss problems and issues that were important to them.

> Informant 07: Well all the times I've been in hospital I've always found the staff excellent. Like helping and they'd talk to you.

However negative experiences were also highlighted where staff appeared too busy, or unwilling to talk or listen to them:

> MF: Did you feel that you could talk to the staff any of them if you felt upset?
>
> Informant 03: No they never had time for a chat with me not the doctors or the nurses, the doctors yeah but that it be once a week, you know. But the nurses were just so busy and flat out they wouldn't really have time. I'm remembering different incidents and thinking back to when I was there. This time it was like they had little cubicle in the middle of the whole hospital and you knock on the door and they sometimes wouldn't even open the door, they were so busy. But you just got the impression maybe it was wrong that they just didn't care like you know or so overworked probably.

They were able to make comparisons between different wards that they had been on and the extent to which there were staff available to talk to them. When they felt that they were ignored anger was expressed.

Physical Amenities

The participants mentioned the physical amenities in the various treatment centres, in relation to their experiences of in-patient care. Their views were mixed as to the helpfulness of these amenities. Food was generally thought to be excellent, in the words of Informant 02:

> I used to really look forward to the meals, the desserts, they'd be like homemade crumbles you know beautiful soups like, really, really nice meals. And you had your menu of course like every day the day before like you could choose what you wanted, and you'd have a choice of five dinners like incredible.

Several participants experienced difficulties in relation to the geography, size and general layout of the wards. Difficulties were experienced in finding their way around the wards. For example as Informant 02 states:

> The first time I was a bit scared really, 'cos it was so big like and I was used to the smallness of [name of private ward] . . . I could never ever figure out the geography of the place. There was one corridor, I just couldn't get it right. I'd go down this way and I'd get to the end and I'd realise no no it should have been the other turn. There was just one turn

that I just, one came back around by the art room and one I don't know
what it is now but I just couldn't get it into my head.

The effect that the decor had was explained by Informant 03:

> But the environment definitely affects people's perceptions of where they
> are, it definitely has knock on effect. You know it's horrible because if
> you're in an environment that's really dull and dark and the TV is always
> on and weird films on the TV.

Some ward areas that had been decorated and furnished for a particular
activity were viewed favourably by the participants. For example a
relaxation room, which had specialised visual effects, was mentioned as
being a place that was conducive to relaxation and promoted positive
feelings in all who went in there. Bedrooms were generally thought to
be nice and cleanliness in most areas was appreciated, but noted particularly when absent.

DISCUSSION OF METHOD

A number of issues emerged in relation to the design of the study and
the approach used. Two of the interviews yielded less data than would
have been desirable. The participants were almost monosyllabic in their
responses, resulting in the researcher having to play more of a role in the
interview than is usually warranted. This could have occurred for a
number of reasons such as nervousness or poor recall. It is suggested,
however, that this was not a problem just for this particular group of
psychiatric patients and could occur in any study using similar methods.
It does not, therefore, invalidate the use of this particular method with
this group, but it suggests that more attention should be paid to sample
selection, in that prior contact with the participants would provide
information on who would yield appropriate information.

During one interview a participant became upset on several occasions
when describing the nature of his mental health problems. The researcher
asked if he wanted to stop and on one occasion the interview was stopped
for a period of time, but the participant requested that it be recommenced.
At the conclusion of the interview the researcher spent some time with
the participant discussing his current emotional difficulties and asked if
he needed further help. The participant declined any further
intervention, but said that although the interview had evoked painful
memories he welcomed the opportunity to tell his story, which might
make a difference to the services being offered to other patients.
Interestingly this response was echoed by many of the other participants.

Some participants tended to move from the discussion topic to their
own particular problems as had occurred in the pilot interview. When

this occurred the researcher had to balance her needs as a researcher against those of the participant. It has been suggested that when this occurs the researcher should attempt to refocus the participant by intervening verbally (Morse and Field, 1995). In some instances, however, the researcher made the decision to allow the participants to talk about the issues that were concerning them as the researcher judged that it would be insensitive to their feelings to indicate a lack of interest in their problems. Refocusing was attempted when it was judged that the participant was ready to return to the topic of the research.

The participants were all aware that the researcher is a psychiatric nurse. At times they referred to this, either by apologising when expressing negative experiences or by asking if the researcher was familiar with members of staff or services that they mentioned. This may have affected in some way the extent of information that they were willing to disclose. It was dealt with in the interview setting by the researcher acknowledging their references but not elaborating or providing any further information as to the nature of her involvement in the services.

While the issues mentioned above must of course be considered, the depth of information imparted by the participants in this study provides justification for the use of phenomenology as a research approach to elicit patients' experiences of care. The sample size in this study was small and further qualitative studies with larger samples are required to build on the findings. Themes generated in this study could be used as the basis for quantitative instruments to explore patients' opinions further on a larger scale.

NOTE

1 Temporary status refers to those patients who are involuntarily detained in hospital under a section of the Mental Treatment Act (1945).

REFERENCES

Burns, N. and Grove, S. (1987) *The Practice of Nursing Research: Conduct, Critique and Utilization*. London: W.I.B. Saunders.
Holloway, I. and Wheeler, S. (1996) *Qualitative Research for Nurses*. London: Blackwell.
Merleau-Ponty, M. (1956) What is phenomenology? *Cross Currents*, 6: 59–70. Cited in Struebert, H.J. and Carpenter, D.R. (eds) (1995) *Qualitative Research in Nursing*. Philadelphia: J.B. Lippincott.
Morse, J.M. (1991) (ed.) *Qualitative Nursing Research*. London: Sage.
Morse, J.M. and Field, P.A. (1995) *Qualitative Research Methods for Health Professionals*. London: Sage.
Sines, D. (1994) The arrogance of power: a reflection on contemporary mental health nursing practice, *Journal of Advanced Nursing*, 20: 894–903.
Spiegleberg, H. (1975) *Doing Phenomenology*. The Hague: Nijhoff. Cited in Struebert, H.J. and Carpenter, D.R. (1995) *Qualitative Research in Nursing: Advancing the Humanistic Perspective*. Philadelphia: J.B. Lippincott.
Streubert, H.J. (1991) Phenomenologic research as a theoretic initiative in community health nursing. *Public Health Nursing*, 8 (2): 119–23.
Streubert, H.J. and Carpenter, D.R. (1995) *Qualitative Research in Nursing: Advancing the Humanistic Perspective*. Philadelphia: J.B. Lippincott.
Van Manen, M. (1984) Practising phenomenological writing, *Phenomenology and Pedagogy*, 2 (1): 36–69.

10

A Study of Irish Women Diagnosed with Breast Cancer

Geraldine McCarthy

INTRODUCTION

In North America and Ireland, one woman in nine will experience breast cancer in her lifetime (Health Canada, 1994; Southern Tumour Register, 1993). In the United Kingdom the figure is one in twelve but increasing (Steel et al., 1992). Breast cancer is therefore of major concern to women. The purpose of this research was to investigate how women respond to, cope with, and adapt to the diagnosis and treatment of breast cancer.

LITERATURE REVIEW

The literature shows that cancer is appraised as stressful and that individuals encountering cancer exhibit a range of psychological responses ranging from confronting reactions to stoic acceptance (Ali and Khalid, 1991; Frank-Stromberg, 1989; Frank-Stromberg et al., 1984; Greer et al., 1979; Knobf, 1994; Krause, 1991; Krause and Krause, 1982; Mishel and Braden, 1988; Morris et al., 1985; Oberst et al., 1989; Pettingale et al., 1985; Wellisch et al., 1996). Most of the studies, however, do not have clearly defined theoretical frameworks. Just one study (Oberst et al., 1989) assessed the degree of harm/loss, threat, challenge associated with cancer as suggested by Lazarus and Folkman (1984). This study was with cancer family-member caregivers. The samples used in the studies on appraisal varied widely in terms of sex, type of cancer, stage of disease, treatment modality, and time since diagnosis. The method used most often was interviews (Frank-Stromborg et al., 1984; Frank-Stromborg, 1989; Krause, 1991; Greer et al., 1979; Mages and Mendlessohn, 1978; Westbrook and Viney, 1982). One longitudinal study (Pettingale et al., 1985) investigated the relationship between appraisal and adjustment to illness in female breast cancer patients. These researchers found significant differences in survival when women were compared by their initial response to cancer suggesting that denial as an initial reaction may be protective and promote survival. A more recent cross-sectional study found that women who perceived control over breast cancer were more likely to use rational strategies and to take an active role during diagnosis, treatment, and recovery (Royak-Schaler, 1992).

Little empirical work has been reported pertaining to the measurement of coping in individuals with cancer and treatment modalities. In the studies reviewed, coping was predominantly measured by interview (Weisman, 1976; Worden and Sobel, 1978; Worden and Weisman, 1977; Ali and Kalid, 1991; Payne, 1990) or semi-structured questionnaires (Gotay, 1984; Lierman, 1988). Just two studies (Perry, 1990; Hertz, 1989) used a coping scale (Jalowiec Coping Scale) to measure coping responses. The studies reported expressions of coping in emotive and cognitive modes ranging from taking firm action, using faith, compliance and information seeking. There is no reported research with breast cancer women using the Lazarus and Folkman Ways of Coping Checklist and none of the studies reviewed used as subjects female breast cancer women who were receiving chemotherapy.

Adjustment to illness has been studied though defined differently in a number of studies both cross-sectional (Krause and Krause, 1982; Baider and Kaplan-DeNour, 1984; Sutherland et al., 1988), longitudinal (Northouse, 1990; Worberg et al., 1989), and a combination of both methods (Penman et al., 1986). Researchers have focused on patients themselves or on the patient and family members, particularly spouses (Baider and Kaplan-DeNour, 1984; Northouse and Swain, 1987; Northouse, 1990). From the literature it is clear that adjustment has been measured in a variety of ways – interviews (Grandstaff, 1976; Jamison et al., 1978; Pettingale et al., 1985), structured questionnaires (Hopkins, 1986), Psychosocial Adjustment to Illness Scale (PAIS) (Baider and Kaplan De-Nour, 1984; Northouse and Swain, 1987; Northouse, 1990; Worberg et al., 1989), the Effect Balance Scale (Northouse and Swain, 1987; Northouse, 1990), the Brief Symptom Inventory (Northouse and Swain, 1987; Northouse, 1990), the Beck Depression Inventory (Krause and Krause, 1982), and Profile of Mood States (Sutherland et al., 1988), a Personality Inventory and the Rotter Internal Locus of Control Scale (Jamison et al., 1978) and with the Bradburns Psychological Well Being Scale (Funch and Mettlin, 1982). Some samples used included individuals with mixed site cancer (Lerman et al., 1990; Krause and Krause, 1982), and were of mixed sex (Lerman et al., 1990; Sutherland et al., 1985). Other samples used husbands and wives (Northouse and Swain, 1987; Northouse, 1990).

Only two of the studies reviewed were based on non USA research – an Israeli study (Baider and Kaplan-DeNour, 1984), which used the

PAIS scale and a Canadian study (Sutherland et al., 1985), which measured mood as an indicator of adjustment. In the literature there is some research reported which uses the PAIS to identify psychosocial adjustment to illness in breast cancer women (Baider and Kaplan De-Nour, 1984; Northouse and Swain, 1987; Northouse, 1990; Wolberg et al., 1989) indicating adjustment problems in emotional, social and vocational dimensions for at least 16 months after diagnosis with cancer. Overall it is difficult to compare findings from studies due to diversity of definitions, operationalisation of concepts and study designs.

A great deal has been learned from the existing research about women's psychosocial responses to breast cancer. The present research seeks to build upon and add to that knowledge base. Gaps in knowledge appear to exist pertaining to appraisal, coping and psychosocial adjustment to cancer and their interrelationships which this research attempts to fill. There is no Irish nursing research with women experiencing breast cancer and neither has other Irish health care research addressed the topic.

CONCEPTUAL FRAMEWORK

The conceptual framework used to investigate the relationship between appraisal of cancer and the person's construction of the experience was derived from Lazarus's and Folkman's theory of stress and coping (Lazarus, 1966; Folkman and Lazarus, 1980; Folkman and Lazarus, 1988b; Folkman et al., 1986). According to this theory, cognitive appraisal is a critical process mediating the person–environment relationship. The underlying theoretical assumption is that 'in order to survive and flourish people must distinguish between benign and dangerous situations' (Lazarus and Folkman, 1984: 19). In the theory the cognitive meanings processed between the events (in this study, the diagnosis and treatment of breast cancer) and the reaction, are the key to understanding the variations among individuals under comparable conditions. However, these distinctions are often subtle, complex, abstract, and dependent on a highly versatile and efficient cognitive system (Lazarus and Folkman, 1984). In this study, hypothesised relationships based on the theoretical framework and between the concepts and their sub-concepts were tested. Specifically, a woman's predominant appraisal of her breast cancer, method of coping, psychosocial adaptation, and demographic/personal aspects were examined for possible relationships (see Figure 1). The study was cross-sectional, descriptive and correlational.

Figure 1. Conceptual Framework used in the Research: Hypothesised relationships between the study variables and measurement instruments used (* Instrument used)

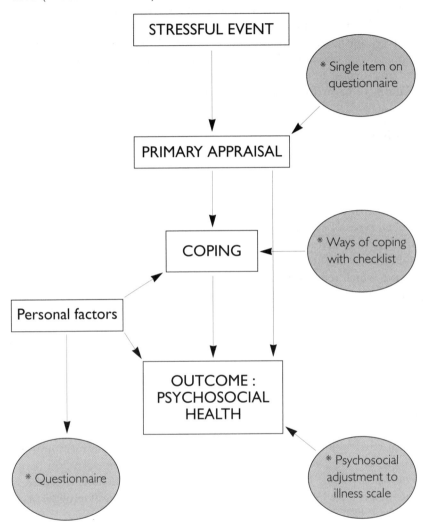

Primary Appraisal

The theoretical definition of primary appraisal used in this study was the meaning that the individual gives to a specific situation. This was based on the theoretical framework of Folkman and Lazarus (1988a). Appraisal was conceptualised as being one in which the cancer represents harm/loss, a potential threat, or challenge (Lazarus and Folkman, 1984). In harm/loss the person considers the damage suffered as irreversible. In threat, harms or losses have not yet occurred but are anticipated. Challenge appraisals are focused on potential for gain or growth inherent in an encounter and are characterized by 'pleasurable emotions such as eagerness, excitement, and exhilaration, whereas threat is centred in potential harms and is characterised by negative emotions such as fear, anxiety, and anger' (Lazarus and Folkman, 1984: 33). For this study, appraisal was operationalised in the answer to questions constructed by the investigator to elicit the meaning of the stressor to the study subject in terms of harm/loss, threat or challenge.

Coping

Coping is theoretically defined as the constantly changing cognitive and behavioural efforts made to master, tolerate or reduce specific external or internal stimuli that are judged to exceed the resources of the individual (Folkman and Lazarus, 1988). Lazarus and Folkman (1984) propose two general types of coping mechanisms: (*a*) problem-focused coping which involves cognitive coping techniques represented by analytic processes and directed at both the environment and self; and (*b*) emotion-focused coping which refers to behaviour-coping effects represented by cognitive manoeuvres or regulation of emotional responses used to change the meaning of situations. This concept was operationalized as the quantitative scores obtained on the Ways of Coping Checklist.

Psychosocial Adjustment

The theoretical definition of psychosocial adjustment was feelings and symptoms of positive mental health and quality of one's reactions to persons, institutions, and other aspects of one's environment. The 'functional efficiencies' demonstrated by an individual in these relationships are highly correlated with his or her levels of psychosocial adjustment (Derogatis, 1986). The operational definition was the quantitative scores obtained on the Psychosocial Adjustment to Illness Scale (Derogatis and Lopez, 1983).

METHOD

Sample

A convenience sample of 86 women newly diagnosed with breast cancer and receiving first time chemotherapy in five oncology outpatient departments attached to university-affiliated hospitals was obtained. Women who met the inclusion criteria were identified by an on-site research assistant in cooperation with the woman's doctor. Participants ranged in age from 26 to 72 years old with a mean of 43.8 years and SD=7.9. Just three individuals were older than 56 years. All women were white and Irish with 80 per cent married and 75 per cent stating that they were housewives and not working outside the home. The time since diagnosis varied from four to 40 weeks, with a mean of 18 weeks. Eighty-eight per cent of the women had received surgical treatment for breast cancer prior to commencing chemotherapy. All participants were receiving similar chemotherapy regimes (CMF) but were at different treatment stages with a mean of six treatments and SD=3 treatments.

Instruments

Appraisal was measured using a researcher constructed forced choice questionnaire, coping with Ways of Coping Checklist (WOCC) (Folkman and Lazarus, 1988), and Adjustment with Derogatis Patient Adjustment to Illness-Self Report Scale (PAIS–SR) (Derogatis, 1986). Demographic information was obtained through the use of a questionnaire developed by the investigator.

Appraisal
The appraisal question was developed by the researcher from Lazarus's and Folkman's (1984) work on appraisal and coping. The three appraisal variables (challenge, threat, and harm/loss) were incorporated into one question and individuals were asked to indicate which best described their most constant feeling. To gain further insight into the participants' interpretation of their own meaning, two further open-ended question were asked.

Ways of Coping Checklist
The WOCC is a 67-item questionnaire containing a wide range of thoughts and actions that people use to deal with internal and/or external demands of specific stressful encounters. For example, the subject reads a statement such as 'looked for the silver lining so to speak . . .' or 'talked to someone to find out more about the situation' and then responded on a 4-point Likert scale in accordance with their use of that particular coping strategy. The coping responses can be classified according to focus (problem-focused or emotion-focused) or as modes of coping in eight separate domains – distancing, seeking support, self-controlling, confronting coping, accepting responsibility, avoidance, problem solving and positive reappraisal.

Psychosocial Adjustment to Illness Scale (PAIS–SR)
The PAIS–SR was developed by Derogatis (1983) to reflect adjustment in seven psychosocial domains, all of which have been shown to have high relevance for adjustment to illness. The seven domains which were assessed by a questionnaire include: health care orientation, vocational environment, domestic environment, sexual relationship, extended family relationship, social environment, and psychological distress. A pilot study supported the use of the instruments without adjustments.

Procedure

One hundred and forty-six newly diagnosed breast cancer patients were identified from the case loads of doctors and asked by an on-site research assistant to participate in the study. An introductory letter stating the purpose of the research and the procedure to be followed was given to the women. Individuals who agreed to participate (n=100) signed a consent form. On the first outpatient visit subjects completed the appraisal questionnaire and on the third (12 weeks later) or subsequent visit completed the Ways of Coping Checklist and the Psychosocial Adjustment to Illness Scale. On average, questionnaires took one/one and a half hours and were completed during the outpatient visit. Those who did not complete the instruments felt too ill, or did not have the energy, concentration or time to do so. Others for a variety of reasons did not continue treatment at the outpatients and were lost to the study.

RESULTS

Appraisal

Answers to the question assessing cognitive appraisal strategies indicated that most women (53 per cent) evaluated the initial diagnosis of breast cancer as 'challenge', followed by 'threat' (37 per cent), and harm-loss (10 per cent). Ninety per cent of respondents choose to use free-text to comment further on their feelings. Fifty per cent of the comments contained the word 'shock' – examples of comments were 'I was initially shocked and angry that this could happen to me and more especially to my husband and family' . . . 'I was totally shocked and devastated' .. and 'at the beginning shock, fear, tears and I felt that God had forgotten about me'. Other comments related to feelings of anger . . . 'I felt angry and sometimes sorry for myself . . .' and 'I felt angry that God should do this to me when I have three young children to look after . . .'. Fewer respondents reported feelings of fear, confusion or anxiety.

Coping

In an effort to test Lazarus's and Folkman's theoretical model (1984) of coping, factor analysis was used to force the variables into two explanatory factors: problem and emotion-focused coping. Once this was done, those variables explaining .55 or greater of the variance in each factor were used to develop a profile score indicating the subject's tendency towards either problem-focused or emotion-focused coping. This score was used to analyse relationships between a subject's overall ways of coping and the other factors in the conceptual framework.

Results showed that individuals used both emotion-focused and cognitive-focused coping strategies with slightly greater use of emotion-focused strategies. To investigate further the use of individual coping strategies which were measured using the different sub-scales, the mean and standard deviation of each subscale were also examined. The strategies most often utilised were 'seeking social support' (x=1.7, SD=0.7), 'distancing' (x=1.5; SD=0.6) and 'positive re-appraisal' (x=1.5; SD=0.7). The least used strategies were 'accepting responsibility' (x=0.7; SD=0.6) and 'confronting the situation' (x=.08, SD=.05)..

Adaptation

Mean responses for the PAIS–SR global scale and for the individual subscales were calculated and correlated with standardised T-scores for a population of patients with mixed types of cancer diagnoses as reported by Derogatis (1990). Global T-scores higher than 62 are positive for clinical levels of psychosocial maladjustment; however, they do not imply a psychiatric disorder (Derogatis, 1990). The sample in this study indicated fairly high scores on the global PAIS (x=54.8; SD=11.7) based on overall norms. This indicated a moderate amount of psychosocial problems. The domains in which scores indicated less adjustment were 'vocational environment' (x=58.4; SD=6.2), and psychological distress (x=58.2, SD=10.4). The domains evidencing the greatest adaptation were 'domestic environment' (x=51.0; SD=8.9) and 'social environment' (x=51.8; SD=14.0).

Appraisal and Coping, Appraisal and Adjustment

The relationship between cognitive appraisal and coping and cognitive appraisal and adjustment was analysed using analysis of variance (ANOVA). Results did not show any significant relationships between the appraisal group and coping scores (problem focused: $F=2.96$, $p=0.06$; emotion focused: $F=0.00$, $p=0.99$). However, significant differences were found

(F=3.57, p=0.03) between the three appraisal groups and psychosocial adjustment to illness. The challenge appraisal group was significantly different from the other two groups with respect to total PAIS scores and in particular with respect to the social environment subscale (F=5.17, p=.007), showing significantly better adjustment in this respect. The latter result should be treated with caution, however, as two appraisal groups contained few participants (harm/loss group N=6, threat group N=31).

Coping and Adaptation

When correlational coefficients were used to examine this relationship no statistically significant associations were found between either problem-focused ($r=-.04$, $p<0.65$) or emotion-focused ($r=0.16$, $p<0.12$) coping strategies and global adaptation (PAIS-SR total scores). A further attempt was made to analyse the relationship between individual coping strategies and psychosocial adjustment to illness. Results showed that less adaptation on the PAIS–SR was related to more 'escape-avoidance' behaviour, a component of emotion-focused coping ($r=.39$, $p<0.00$). Use of escape-avoidance behaviour also correlated significantly with the 'health orientation' ($r=.29$), 'domestic environment' ($r=.36$), 'sexual relations' ($r=.29$), 'extended family' ($r=.36$), 'social environment' ($r=.42$) and 'psychosocial distress' ($r=.29$) scales. In all cases, significance levels were $p<0.01$.

Other Findings

Using Pearson's correlation statistics, several statistically significant relationships were found between demographic or medical variables and the WOCC and PAIS–SR scales. Age was found to be related to the sexual relations sub-scale ($r=.22$, $p<0.05$). Time since diagnosis was found to be significantly related to the sexual relations sub-scale ($r=.24$, $p<0.04$), and *inversely* ($r=-.24$, $p<0.04$) related to social support ($r=-.28$, $p< 0.01$), and number of chemotherapy treatments was significantly related to social support ($r=-.26$, $p<.01$) and to the self controlling sub-scale in the WOCC ($r=-.23$, $p<.02$).

DISCUSSION

Results indicating that women with cancer predominantly perceived their situation as either a challenge (n=47) or anticipated threat (n=31) supports the work of Lazarus and Folkman (1984). Similar findings were also reported by Frank-Stromborg (1989) in a study of 461 male and female mixed cancer patients within six months of diagnosis when 45 per cent of the sample reported confrontive behaviour. The same researcher (Frank-Stromborg et al.) in 1984 found that 27 per cent of 340 mixed cancer patients reported feelings of challenge when confronted with cancer. However, in these studies the interview was used exclusively to determine the appraisal strategies used.

The challenge group in this study could be considered those who desire mastery or control over the situation. In the Irish culture and in a country where religious beliefs and family norms are strong, people are admired for maintaining a stiff upper lip in the face of adversity. Results showing that the majority of women found the situation one of challenge was not therefore surprising. Subjects were also given an opportunity to describe their feelings in their own words. Ninety per cent of participants choose free text to comment and 50 per cent of the comments contained the word 'shock' or 'anger'. Fewer respondents wrote about feelings of fear, devastation, fright, confusion, and anxiety. The self reporting of shock as a primary feeling is similar to the results of a Finnish study (Krause, 1991) which reported that 68 per cent of the 123 mixed cancer sample reported feelings of shock when confronted with the diagnosis of cancer. Further studies with American samples also show similar findings (Cantor, 1978; Frank-Stromborg, 1989; Holland and Mastrvitor, 1976; Mishel and Baiden, 1988; Weisman et al., 1980). An interesting finding was that the feelings expressed in free text did not emulate those expressed in the forced choice question on cognitive appraisal. However, the differences in answers could be caused by both questions being interpreted in different ways. Because the choices offered in the appraisal question may not be mutually exclusive a more useful approach to assess appraisal might be a multiple item scale to measure the three dimensions of challenge, harm/loss and anticipated threat. Alternatively an interview may be useful for the investigation of cognitive appraisal.

Results show that both problem-focused and emotion-focused coping strategies were used by the sample with emotion-focused coping responses used slightly more often. These findings agree with results from a study of stressful encounters in middle-aged men and women (Folkman and Lazarus, 1980) and an investigation pertaining to how college students cope with examination stress (Folkman et al., 1986). The seemingly contradictory forms of coping used suggest that individuals during the course of a stressful encounter alternate the use of coping strategies. Based on their research Folkman and Lazarus (1988b) propose that problem-focused coping is used more often in encounters that were appraised as changeable and emotion-focused coping in encounters seen as unchangeable. As the patients in this study used slightly more emotion-focused coping strategies it could be suggested that they saw the situation as unchangeable, a high stake situation, or one in which they had few options. Lazarus and Folkman (1984) suggest that when levels of stress increase greatly, the individual's ability to perform problem-focused coping diminishes. Thus the individual reliance on emotion-focused coping increases. It is interesting to note that at the commencement of the study doctors and nurses involved in this research commented on their perception relating to high stress levels in patients. They suggested that stress be studied in parallel with coping. Further research on the topic of coping with breast cancer may benefit from a concurrent investigation of patient stress.

When particular domains of coping were investigated the strategies used most often were seeking social support, positive reappraisal, distancing, and planful problem solving. Seeking social support is defined by Folkman and Lazarus (1988) as having components of both emotion-focused and problem-focused coping strategies. Particular actions which were undertaken were 'talked to someone to find out more about the situation', and 'accepted sympathy and understanding from someone'. The use of 'accepting sympathy and understanding' is indicative of emotion-focused social support. This finding is important and may benefit from a qualitative investigation. Positive reappraisal (a problem-focused coping strategy) was the second most used coping mechanism. 'Rediscovered what is important in life' was the item most often chosen as representing this strategy. This points to self reflection and working in an effort to find meaning in the situation. In prior studies (Folkman et al., 1988), problem-focused coping and positive reappraisal were highly correlated. Similar findings were present in this study. This suggests that positive reappraisal may help problem-focused forms of coping. Distancing was the third most used coping strategy and is considered by Folkman and Lazarus (1984) as emotion-focused coping. Distancing describes efforts to detach oneself from the situation. It could be suggested that if an individual were to use this form of coping predominantly instead of attending to the particular situation, the outcome might be unfavourable. However the strategy might be adaptive to an outcome if it were seen as unalterable and as such it might help the individual.

The research asked if the type of appraisal expressed by subjects significantly influenced coping strategies. Persons who appraised the situation as a challenge rather than a threat were hypothesised to differ from those who appraised it in other ways. No statistical differences were found between the women comprising the three appraisal groups with respect to emotion-focused or problem-focused coping strategies. This finding was unexpected, as for Folkman et al. (1986a and b) coping was strongly related to cognitive appraisal. However, in their studies appraisal was measured predominantly through interviews. These findings may have been affected by the study design.

Results indicated that some disruption in psychosocial adjustment occurred particularly in vocational environment, psychological distress, extended family relationships and sexual relations domains. The results are similar to those of other studies (Baider and Kaplan-DeNour, 1984; Friedman et al., 1988; Gilbar and Kaplan-DeNour, 1988; Northouse and Swain, 1987; Northouse and Swain, 1987; Northouse, 1990; Worberg et al., 1989). However, the sample in this study shows poorer adjustment than that in a study of adaptation to diabetes mellitus by White et al. (1992).

In this study the overall relationship between primary appraisal and outcome expressed in the Psychosocial Adjustment to Illness scale was weak. This finding was unexpected as it was hypothesised that there would be substantial differences between individuals who perceived the disease as a challenge versus an anticipated threat. Methodological difference or sampling may have accounted for this. Other factors which may have influenced the results may relate to preparation for treatment or the network of support which surrounded these women. Little research exists in cancer populations explaining the relationship between coping and adjustment to illness. The results in this study showed no statistically significant relationships between problem-focused or emotion-focused coping styles and the total PAIS scores. Because problem-focused coping strategies are perceived to be more adaptive and reality oriented, the expectation was that they would provide higher adjustment. However, contrary to expectation, problem-focused coping did not have a direct relationship with psychosocial adjustment to illness. This is difficult to explain as previous studies (De Maio-Esteves, 1990; Folkman et al., 1986a; Folkman et al., 1986b) linked problem-focused coping with adjustment and positive health outcomes and emotion-focused coping behaviour with poor adjustment and poor health outcomes (McCarthy Neundorfer, 1991). Individuals who had poorer psychosocial adjustment to illness used more escape-avoidance behaviour and less of the coping strategy of distancing. This finding is consistent with Felton et al.'s (1984) results involving psychological adjustment of adults with hypertension, diabetes mellitus, cancer, and arthritis.

CONCLUSION

Overall this study identified situation specific information on cognitive appraisal, coping responses, social support and psychosocial adjustment to illness in Irish women with breast cancer. As choices had to be made about the sample, design and measurement of variables the study had certain limitations including convenience sample, self selection, cross-sectional design, instrumentation, self reporting and social desirability of response. A study using a different measure of appraisal may be useful and studies with samples from other countries should prove interesting. A longitudinal investigation is also required to monitor ongoing relationships over time.

The study has provided insight into women's reactions to and perceptions of breast cancer. The Folkman and Lazarus stress and coping framework provided a theoretical perspective for the study. In the absence of similar reported studies on women with breast cancer receiving chemotherapy, or in literature pertaining to cognitive appraisal, coping and psychological outcomes in a cancer population, this study not only complements the work of Folkman and Lazarus but also makes an important contribution to nursing knowledge in general and Irish nursing in particular.

REFERENCES

Ali, Nagia, S. and Khalid, H. (1991) Identification of stressors, level of stress, coping strategies, and coping effectiveness among Egyptian mastectomy patients, *Cancer Nursing*, 14 (5): 232–9.

Baider, L. and Kaplan-DeNour, A. (1984) Couples' reactions and adjustment to mastectomy: A preliminary report. *International Journal of Psychiatry in Medicine*, 14(3): 265–76.

Cantor, R.C. (1978) *And Time to Live: Towards Emotional Well Being During the Crisis of Cancer*. New York: Harper & Row.

Cassileth, B.R., Zupkis, R.V, Sutton-Smith, K., and Mach, V. (1984) Information and participation preferences among cancer patients, *Annals of Internal Medicine*, 92: 832–6.

De-Maio-Esteves, M. (1990) Mediators of daily stress and perceived health status in adolescent girls, *Nursing Research*, 39 (6): 340–46.

Department of Health (1991) Health Statistics, Dublin: Department of Health.

Derogatis, L.R. (1986) The psychosocial adjustment to illness scale (PAIS), *Journal of Psychometric Research*, 30: 77–91.

Derogatis, L.R. and Lopez, H.C. (1983) *The Psychosocial Adjustment to Illness Scale: Administration, Scoring and Procedures Manual*. Baltimore: Clinical Psychometric Research.

Derogatis, L.R. and Spencer, P.M. (1982) *The Brief Symptom Inventory: Administration, Scoring and Procedures Manual*. Baltimore: Clinical Psychometric Research.

Felton, B.J., Revenson, T.A., and Hinrichsen, G.A. (1984) Stress and coping in the explanation of psychologic adjustment among chronically ill adults, *Social Science Medicine*, 18: 889–98.

Folkman, S. (1984) Personal control and stress and coping processes: a theoretical analysis. *Journal of Personality and Social Psychology*, 46: 839–52.

Folkman, S. and Lazarus, R.S. (1980) An analysis of coping in a middle age community sample, *Journal of Health and Social Behaviour*, 21 (30): 219–39.

Folkman, S. and Lazarus, R.S. (1988a) *Manual for the Ways of Coping Questionnaire*. Palo Alto: Consulting Psychologists Press.

Folkman, S. and Lazarus, R.S. (1988b) Coping as a mediator of emotion, *Journal of Personality and Social Psychology*, 54 (3): 466–75.

Folkman, S., Lazarus, R., Dunkel-Schetter, C., DeLongis, A., and Gruen, R. (1986a) The dynamics of a stressful encounter: cognitive appraisal, coping, and encounter outcomes, *Journal of Personality and Social Psychology*, 50: 992–1003.

Folkman, S., Lazarus, R., Gruen, R.J., and DeLongis, A. (1986b) Appraisal, coping, health status and psychological adjustment symptoms, *Journal of Personality and Social Psychology*, 50 (3): 571–79.

Frank-Stromborg, M. (1989) Reaction to the diagnosis of cancer questionnaire: Development and psychometric evaluation, *Nursing Research*, 38 (6): 364–69.

Frank-Stromborg, M., Wright, P.S., Segale, M., and Diermann, J. (1984) Psychological impact of the cancer diagnosis, *Oncology Nursing Forum*, 11 (3): 16–23.

Friedman, L.C., Brae, P.E., Nelson, D.V., Lane, M., Smith, F.E., and Dworkin, R.J. (1988) Women with breast cancer: perceptions of family functioning and adjustment to illness, *Psychosomatic Medicine*, 50 (3): 529–40.

Funch, D.P. and Mettlin, C. (1982) The role of support in relation to recovery from breast surgery, *Social Science and Medicine*, 16: 91–98.

Gilbar, O. and Kaplan-DeNour, A.K. (1988) Adjustment to illness and dropout in chemotherapy, *Journal of Psychosomatic Medicine*, 50 (3): 529–40.

Gotay, C. (1984) The experience of cancer during early and advanced stages: the views of patients and their mates, *Social Science Medicine*, 18 (17): 605–13.

Grandstaff, N. (1976) The impact of breast cancer on the family. in J. Vaeth (ed.), *Breast Cancer: Its Impact on the Patient, Family, and Community*. Basel: Karger.

Greer, S., Morris, T. and Pettingale, K.W. (1979) Psychological response to breast cancer: Effect on outcome. *Lancet*, 2: 785–7.

Health Canada (1994) *Report National Forum on Breast Cancer*. Ottawa: Health Canada.

Hertz, K. (1989) The Relationship between level of hope and level of coping and other variables in patients with cancer, *Oncology Nursing Forum*, 16 (1): 67–72.

Holland, J.C. and Mastrvitor, R. (1980) Psychological adaptation to breast cancer, *Cancer*, 46:1042–5.

Hopkins M.B. (1986) Information seeking and adaptation outcomes in women receiving chemotherapy for breast cancer, *Cancer Nursing*, 9 (5): 256–62.

Jamison, K.R., Wellisch, D.K., and Pasnau, R.O. (1978) Psychosocial aspects of mastectomy 1. The woman's perspective, *American Journal of Psychiatry*, 135: 432–36.

Knobf, M.T. (1994) Decision making for primary breast cancer treatment, MedSurg, *Nursing*, 3 (3), 169–75.

Krause, K. (1991) Contracting cancer and coping with it: patients' experiences, *Cancer Nursing*, 14 (5): 240–5.

Krause, K. (1993) Coping with Cancer, *Western Journal of Nursing Research*, 15 (1): 31–43.

Krause, H.J.and Krause, J.H. (1982) Cancer as crisis: the critical elements of adjustment, *Nursing Research*, 31 (2): 96–101.

Lazarus, R. (1966) *Psychological stress and the coping process*. New York: McGraw Hill.

Lazarus, R., and Folkman, S. (1984) *Stress, Appraisal and Coping*. New York: Springer.

Lerman, C., Rimer, B., Blumberg, B., Cristinzio, S., Engstrom, P.E., MacElwee, N., O Connor, K., and Seay, J. (1990) Effects of coping style and relaxation on cancer chemotherapy side effects and emotional responses, *Cancer Nursing*, 13(5): 308–15.

Lierman, J. (1988) Discovery of breast changes: Woman's response and nursing implications. *Cancer Nursing*, 2(6): 352–62.

Mages, N.L. and Mendelssohn, G.A. (1978) Effects of cancer on patients lives: a personological approach, in: G.C. Stone, F. Cohen and N.E. Adler (eds), *Health Psychology – A Handbook*. San Francisco: Jossey Bass.

McCarthy Neundorfer, M. (1991) Coping and health outcomes in spouse caregivers of persons with dementia, *Nursing Research*, 40 (5): 260–6

Mishel, M.H., and Braden, C.J. (1988) Finding meaning: antecedents of uncertainty in illness, *Nursing Research*, 37: 98–103.

Morris, T., Blake, S., and Buckley, M. (1985) Development of a method for rating cognitive response to the diagnosis of cancer, *Social Science and Medicine*, 20: 795–802.

Morris, T., Greer, S., and Haybittle, J. (1985) Predictors of psychosocial adjustment in patients newly diagnosed with gynaecological cancer, *Cancer Nursing*, 7: 291–00.

Northouse, L, (1990) Longitudinal study of the adjustment of patients and husbands to breast cancer, *Oncology Nursing Forum*, 17(3): 39–45.

Northouse, L.L. (1989) A longitudinal study of the adjustment of patients and husbands to breast cancer. *Oncology Nursing Forum*, 16: 511–16.

Northouse, L., Cracchiolo-Caraway, Appel, C.P. (1991), Psychological consequences of breast cancer on partner and family, *Seminars in Oncology Nursing*, 7(3): 216–23.

Northouse, L.L. and Swain, M.A. (1987) Adjustment of patients and husbands to the initial impact of breast cancer. *Nursing Research*, 36 (4): 221–25

Oberst, M.T., Gass, K.A. and Ward, S.E. (1989) Caregiving demands and appraisal of stress among family caregivers. *Cancer Nursing*, 12(4): 209–15.

Penman, D.T., Bloom, J.R., Fotopoulos, S., Cook, M.R., Holland, J.C., Gates, C., Flamer, D., Murawski, B., Ross, R., Brandt, U., Muenz, L.R., and Pee, D. (1986) The impact of mastectomy on self-concept and social function: a combined cross-sectional and longitudinal study with comparison groups, *Women and Health*, 11(3/4): 101–30.

Perry, G.R. (1990) Loneliness and coping among tertiary-level adult cancer patients in the home. *Cancer Nursing*, 13 (3): 167–75.

Pettingale, K., Morris, T., Greer, S. and Haybittle, J. (1985) Mental attitudes to cancer: An additional prognostic factor. *Lancet*, 1: 750–753.

Pettingale, K.W., Philalithis, A., Tee, D.E.A., and Greer, H.E. (1981) The biological correlates of psychological responses to breast cancer, *Journal of Psychosomatic Research*, 25: 453–58.

Royak-Schaler, R. (1992) Psychological processes in breast cancer: a review of selected research, *Journal of Psychological Oncology*, 9(4): 71–89.

Southern Tumour Register, (1993) *11th Annual Report*. Cork: University College.

Steel, C.M., Cohen, B., and Porter, D. (1992) Familial breast cancer, *Seminal Cancer Biology*, 3 (3): 141–50.

Sutherland, H.J., Walker P., and Till, J.E. (1988) The development of a method for determining oncology patients emotional distress using linear analogue scale, *Cancer Nursing*, 11 (5): 303–8.

Weisman, A.D., Worden, J.W., and Sobel, H.J. (1980) *Psychosocial Screening and Interventions with Cancer Patients*. Cambridge, Mass: Authors.

Weisman, A. (1976) Early diagnosis of vulnerability in cancer patients. *American Journal of Medical Science*, 271: 187–96.

Wellisch, D.K., Schains, W., Gritz, E.R., and Wang, H. (1996) Psychological functioning of daughters of breast cancer patients, Part III: Experiences and perceptions of daughters related to mothers' breast, *Psycho-Oncology*, 5 (3), 271–81.

Westbrook, M. and Viney, L. (1982) Psychological reactions to the onset of chronic illness, *Social Science in Medicine*, 16, 889–905.

White, N.E., Richter, J.M. and Fry, C. (1992) Coping, social support and adaptation to chronic illness, *Western Journal of Nursing Research*, 14(2): 211–24.

Worberg, W.H., Tanner, M.A., Malee, J.F. and Romsaas, E.P. (1989) Psychosexual adaptation to breast cancer surgery, *Cancer*, 63 (8): 1645–55.

Worden, J.W. and Sobel, H.J. (1978) Ego strength and psychosocial adaptation to cancer, *Psychomatic Medicine*, 40: 585–92.

Worden, J.W. and Weisman, A.D. (1977) The fallacy in post mastectomy depression. *American Journal of Medical Science*, 273: 169–75

11
The Role of the Professional General Nurse

Aine O'Meara Kearney

INTRODUCTION

The health services are currently undergoing rapid change. Emphasis on the provision of cost-effective and efficient services challenge all healthcare workers to justify their contribution to patient care. In Ireland, how nurses perceive their role and the foundations upon which that role may be articulated in the future have not been subject to empirical enquiry. This study was designed to describe the role of the general nurse.[1]

BACKGROUND

The evolution of nursing has waxed and waned over the centuries and has been heavily influenced by the beliefs and values of society. The impact of religious orders is notable in that care of the sick and vulnerable has traditionally been viewed as part of the Christian ethos. Gavin (1997) adds that the influence of groups, notably medical doctors, who have a vested interest in nursing's development, have also served to shape the nature of nursing practice.

Contemporary writers focus on nursing as a professional discipline. According to Kenney (1995: 3), a professional discipline is 'identified by a specific field of enquiry and the shared values and beliefs of its members about its social commitment and the nature of its service'. The shift in status from a vocational occupation to a professional discipline is largely attributable to nurse educationalists in the USA who, challenged to think about the art and the science of nursing, sought to explicate a conceptual definition of the role of the nurse and how that role could be operationalised.

In practice, the extent to which theory has influenced the delivery of patient care is variable. *The Value of Nursing* (Royal College of Nursing

(RCN), 1992) appears to present a picture of a professional body whose aims and goals are unified, with patient care delivery occurring in partnership with patients and delivered by autonomous and accountable nurses. White (1988) disputes this assumption and suggests the presence of three distinguishable subgroups in nursing – the managers (who control staff and maintain the status quo), the generalists (who see nursing as a job and are task orientated) and the professionalists (patient-centred, autonomous and accountable nurses). In addition, there is evidence to support the assumption that nursing care is not always commensurate with patient need or expectation, particularly with regard to continuity of care delivery and interpersonal skills (Moores and Thompson, 1986; Astedt Kurki and Haggman-Laitila, 1992; Weston et al., 1995; McColl et al., 1996). Furthermore, while role development and specialisation appear to have become pathways for autonomous practice and extension of role boundaries in the USA, a different picture emerges elsewhere. In the UK, role extension appears to be focused on the delegation of clinical tasks that previously consumed the more expensive time of medical doctors (Richardson and Maynard, 1995). Expanded roles appear to be associated with role ambiguity, role conflict and role stress (Bousfield, 1997; Hicks and Hennessy, 1998). In Ireland, advanced practitioner role development has been largely unstructured. While the Interim Report (Commission on Nursing, 1997) met with many nurses who called themselves 'specialists', a lack of role coherence was manifest.

Various forces serve to threaten the future role of the professional nurse. Demographic, social and technical changes are shaping future directions in healthcare delivery. Meanwhile, the commercial management styles of various healthcare organisations and their emphasis on efficient resource utilisation have led to a close scrutiny of nurses and their contribution to healthcare services. Contemporary studies in the UK (DHSS, 1986; DHSS, 1988) have proposed the dilution of the richness of the nursing skill mix in order to achieve fiscal management objectives. To date, however, there is a lack of empirical evidence to support the cost-effectiveness of nursing skill-mix dilution (Minyard et al., 1986; Donovan and Lewis, 1987; Helt and Jelinek, 1988). Furthermore, there is tentative support in the literature for the view that the quality of the nursing service is proportional to the level of competence of the person providing the service (Hinshaw et al., 1981; Pearson et al., 1987; Davies, 1992; Carr-Hill et al., 1992). What studies on skill mix do highlight, however, is the high proportion of non-nursing duties undertaken by nurses (DHSS, 1988; Ball et al., 1989; Chang, 1995). This finding gives tentative support to the need for a helper grade to assist the professional nurse. Ironically, there is a lack of agreement among nurses regarding the duties a helper grade should assume (DHSS, 1988; Chang, 1995).

Recent educational reform has paved the way for the introduction of another non-nursing grade – the support worker. While in theory nurses were to control support worker practices, in reality this appears not to have occurred. There is evidence of a handover of professional tasks to the support worker group (Thornley, 1997) and a consequent perception that support workers may be eroding the boundaries of nursing practice (Bradshaw, 1996/1997).

The impasse nursing finds itself in raises questions with respect to its future. The need for nurses to define their role and contribution to patient care clearly has never been greater. In Ireland, while anecdotal evidence suggests concern exists among nurse professionals regarding the future of nursing (Savage, 1997), the role of the professional nurse has not been subject to empirical enquiry. This study was designed to address this deficit. It was anticipated that such a study could inform and guide future developments in nursing in Ireland.

AIM OF THE STUDY

The aim of this pilot study was to gain a conceptual description of the role of Irish professional general nurses, as perceived by general nurses themselves.

RESEARCH DESIGN

A qualitative approach using a grounded theory design was used in this pilot study. Rationale for selection of this approach was based on the need to gain a whole picture from the actor's perspective which 'transcends the bits and pieces' (Lo-Biondo-Wood and Haber, 1994: 257). Symbolic interactionism, the philosophical foundation for grounded theory, is integrally linked to the concept of role and how individuals determine appropriate role behaviours. As the aim of this pilot study was to conceptualise the processes underpinning the nursing role, a grounded theory design appeared appropriate.

Grounded theory is designed to propose or develop a theoretical explanation for the psychological and social realities in the substantive area under study. An essential element of this methodology is that data collection and analysis occur simultaneously. Two methodological techniques are essential to the process of developing theory that is grounded: the constant comparative method and theoretical sampling (Glaser and Strauss, 1967). The constant comparative method involves the researcher making constant comparisons for similar and deviant incidents throughout a complex coding process. In open coding, the data are broken down into discrete parts to identify incidents. Similar codes are grouped together according to their 'fit' into categories. Categories are further developed in terms of their properties and dimensions. Axial coding is directed towards relating subcategories to a category and categories to each other. Glaser (1992) supports the selective use of various coding families to sensitise the researcher to possible linkages between categories and subcategories. Strauss and Corbin (1990) also recommend the use of a coding paradigm around one category at a time. Final modification and integration is guided by a process called selective coding. The aim is to discover the core category or the basic social psychological process. Conditions, strategies and consequences that relate to the core category and that validate the relationship between categories and the core category are verified.

Theoretical sampling is integrally linked with the constant comparative method. According to Strauss and Corbin (1990: 176) it involves 'sampling on the basis of concepts that have proven and theoretical relevance to the evolving theory'. Thus, participant selection is determined by the emerging concepts, dimensions and variations. The aim is to select participants who can further elucidate the substantive area under study. The techniques of constant comparison and theoretical sampling continue until no additional data evolve (theoretical saturation) and the theory is rich, full and complete (Morse, 1995).

DATA COLLECTION

Focus group interviews were used to generate data. Basch (1987: 411) defines the focus group as an 'approach to learning about population subgroups with respect to conscious, semi-conscious and unconscious psychological and social characteristics and processes'. As social or communication events (Albrecht et al., 1993), focus groups are not concerned with consensus building, rather they seek to explore all participants' various experiences and feelings on a topic within a dynamic, discursive environment. The aim of the moderator is to gain insight into the dynamic relationships of beliefs and values and how these beliefs and values relate to current and projected human behaviour and activity (Folch-Lyon and Trost, 1981). An interview guide, which identifies areas to be explored during the course of interviews, is used.

The main advantage of focus group interviews is that they allow the researcher to gather data from a number of participants simultaneously. Hansler and Cooper (1986) further suggest that the security of 'being in a crowd' frequently leads to greater disclosure and a more candid portrayal of reality. While some researchers suggest that group participants should be homogeneous and have no previous relationships with each other, Morgan (1992) argues that, in organisations, this is not possible nor often desirable. Homogeneity can be enhanced, though, by seeking group members who are cohesive in terms of their social standing and backgrounds. Typically, each focus group comprises 4–12 participants (Basch, 1987; Krueger, 1988). The number of focus groups is determined by saturation of information. A minimum of four groups is suggested (Nyamathi and Shuler, 1990).

Gaining Access

The pilot study was conducted in a large regional hospital in Ireland. The hospital includes a general nurse training school and, in partnership with a third-level institution, provides for a diploma programme of nurse education and training. The researcher wrote to the Director of Nursing to seek permission to undertake the pilot study. She subsequently met with the Director of Nursing in order to present a broad outline of the study, including the methods of data collection and analysis to be used. Consent to undertake the study was obtained.

Determining Group Participants

The criteria for inclusion in the study were that all participants be RGNs, either directly or indirectly involved in the care of acute medical/surgical patients in wards which had experienced changes in their skill mix as a result of the introduction of the Diploma programme of nurse education and training. Nurses who had worked abroad in the previous five years or who had been employed in the hospital for less than two years were excluded.

The researcher made known the aims and objectives of her study to a wide population of nurses in the hospital and invited nurses interested in participating to contact her directly. This method of invitation was chosen to reduce selection bias and also to ensure no candidate felt coerced to participate. Sampling was guided by theoretical sampling. Thus, while an initial cohort of ward sisters was selected, subsequent group selection was determined by the emerging hypotheses and the number of interviews conducted was a function of theoretical completeness. A minimum of one week's notice was given of all focus group interviews.

A pre-test facilitated the researcher in gaining confidence in data collection and analysis. It also provided a valuable opportunity to reflect on the experience of acting as moderator to a focus group interview.

Conducting the Interviews

Interviews were conducted in a private office within the hospital complex where the risk of interruptions was minimal. Prior to commencing each interview, a full explanation of the aims of the study and the research design was given to all participants. The issue of confidentiality was discussed and the researcher's and participants' role in upholding this criterion agreed. Participants were also made aware of their freedom to withdraw from the study at any time. To offset the potential risk of peer pressure to comply with dominant views, the researcher explained to each group that all views merited equal weight and thus were of value to the research. Participants were then invited to sign a consent form, indicating their voluntary participation in the study.

An interview guide was used. In keeping with the recommendations of Kingry et al. (1990), each focus group interview started with a general introductory question in order to encourage all participants to contribute to the conversation. Open-ended questions were posed. As interviews progressed, the researcher asked participants to clarify issues that emerged during the process of group interaction. Consistent with theoretical sampling, some alterations were made to the interview guide as analysis progressed. Interviews became more focused as conceptual codes and categories emerged from the data and various hypotheses were tested. All interviews (n=4×4) lasted between one and one and a half hours and were tape recorded.

In order to ensure that the researcher would not influence emerging data, she refrained from offering opinions or answering questions during the course of focus group interviews. A field journal was kept in which the researcher recorded her own personal reflections of the researcher role and the dynamics of group interactions. Emerging patterns and concepts which merited further investigation were also noted.

DATA ANALYSIS

Data were transcribed verbatim within 72 hours of each focus group interview. Transcription included information on pauses and gaps, as well as comments in brackets detailing emotional tones. Transcripts were then read by the researcher while listening to the tapes. This served to improve familiarity with and absorption of data, while verifying accuracy of transcriptions. A duplicate copy of interview transcripts was made. One copy was kept in safe keeping, the other was used for analysis.

A line by line analysis of the data occurred in order to discover and name concepts which reflected the substance of the data. Where possible, participants' words were used to code concepts. This helped to ensure the researcher did not assign her own meaning to data. These code words were written in the wide margins of the transcripts for easy retrieval. Similar concepts were then grouped together to form categories. Properties and dimensions were sought through a constant re-examination of data and in subsequent interviews. The paradigm model was used to investigate causal conditions, context, action and consequences of categories. Relationships between categories began to emerge. As higher order categories evolved, they were returned to the data and interviews to be tested. The researcher also returned to the literature in order to link the emerging theory with research which supported or refuted it. Data collection and analysis, using the constant comparison method continued until theoretical saturation occurred.

Throughout the process of coding and analysis, theoretical notes were written down as memos on index cards, as well as the incident which precipitated the idea. These memos were cross referenced with the transcripts for easy retrieval. As categories emerged, memos were sorted according to categories. Linkages between memos served to facilitate development of linkages between categories and often revealed areas that required further exploration. In the final phase of analysis, categories were integrated with the core category and each other to develop a story line which explained the role of the general nurse.

RIGOUR

The themes 'credibility', 'applicability', consistency' and 'confirmability' are proposed as the criteria for judging the scientific rigour of qualitative research (Guba and Lincoln, 1981; Sandelowski, 1986). In order to enhance rigour in this pilot study, several measures were undertaken. The aim of the study was stated and the decision trail used by the researcher is clearly outlined. A detailed line by line analysis of data was undertaken in order to ensure the emergent theory 'fit' the data. The process of theoretical sampling and the formulation of inclusion criteria both served to reduce selection bias. A significant degree of agreement was achieved between the researcher's codes and those of an independent expert for the first focus group interview. Following a detailed analysis, findings were returned to eleven participants for verification. Agreement of the emergent theory by these participants was obtained.

FINDINGS

From an extensive process of analysis, three major processes or conceptual categories emerged which describe the role of the general nurse: developing interactive–supportive relationships, knowledgeable care-giving, and pulling everything together. It was found that the intervening variables of workload, education and operational policies served to mediate or influence these processes. The core category, working against the odds to move nursing forward, encapsulates role reality or the psychological social process of being a general nurse.

Developing Interactive–Supportive Relationships

Developing interactive–supportive relationships describes the affective aspect of being a general nurse. Nurses described themselves as the professionals who cared for patients most directly for the longest period of time.

> I think a patient's care can transfer through various stages of say physio-therapy, medical support, social worker support. But the nurse is there all the time, from start to finish, be it from admission to discharge, you're there through all the stages. (G1, P2)

This consistency was deemed to put nurses in a unique position to develop supportive interactive relationships with patients. Indeed, effective nurse-patient relationships were considered the foundation upon which high quality nursing care delivery could be achieved.

> Most of the time, when you know you're being effective, it's really when you're interacting interpersonally with someone. (G4, P3)

Nurses recounted a hierarchy of patient need for integration and support and described various strategies used to move patients forward, some-times in adverse conditions. When therapeutically effective relationships were established, it was stated that patients showed confidence and trust in nurses and frequently confided in them. Nurses in turn reported advocating on behalf of patients. This frequently materialised into being ready to 'stick your neck out' or 'bend the truth slightly'.

A number of factors were found to militate against the development of effective relationships with patients. Some nurses reported a lack of education in communication skills. Consequently there was a fear of saying something that 'will catch up on you later' (G3, P4). In addition, family decisions to withhold information from patients were perceived to create barriers in communication, while constraints on information giving regarding diagnosis were seen to promote unequal nurse–patient relationships. Ironically, it was reported that some doctors constructed their information giving carefully so as not to invite questions. Consequently, nurses often ended up picking up the pieces after them.

Heavy workloads were reported as a major prohibitive factor in developing interactive supportive relationships. Nurses reported being constantly interrupted when interacting with patients and that patients appeared to sense when they were under pressure.

> If you're busy, the first thing I find the patient will say to you is have you no help today or tonight or whatever? Are you on your own? And I might say, oh, I'll be fine. In an hour the relief will be here. But that puts them under pressure. They're thinking of you because you're on your own or you're under pressure or whatever or you're short staff. And they lose a little bit of confidence then too. They may need you but they hold back. (G2, P1)

Consequently, it would appear that the necessary time and manpower were not always available to build up trusting relationships with patients. Nurses expressed frustration that patients were not getting the attention they deserved. This was interfering with the nurses' ability to gain a whole picture of the patient and was thus compromising holistic care delivery. Nurses also sensed it left patients feeling vulnerable. It was also stated that operational policies such as bed closures and bed transfers appeared to be largely driven by financial concerns. These factors were having a major impact on care provision.

> I think in the last year the bed situation and transfer is just dreadful. I can give you lists of . . . er, there's one particular patient who came in for a simple thyroid and ended in five different beds in 24 hours and she didn't, I mean, every time she woke, there was a different nurse looking after her and she was on a different floor. (G2, P2)

Meanwhile, patients were venting their anger and frustration at the system on nurses, who reported feeling vulnerable, demoralised and powerless to effect any change due to lack of management support.

Knowledgeable Care Giving

Knowledgeable care giving is the category that describes the extent to which nurses use their knowledge and skill in caring for patients and in moving patients' health forward. Nurses spoke about a greater emphasis on the holistic assessment and planning of care.

> I think our assessing and planning is more effective now, you know, we wouldn't do it properly before. Whereas now I do feel most people really do go in and plan what they're going to do for a patient, from every aspect, you know. (G3, P4)

Knowing the significance of various observations and being able to equate these observations to the patient's medical condition was deemed important. Being educated also empowered nurses to act as health educators, a role they valued and felt patients expected. It further appeared to direct care giving.

> We have to think about what we are doing as well. You're not just doing something for the sake of doing it, because that's the way it was always done (G3, P2)

Many nurses felt their knowledge and assessment skills were the key criteria which distinguished the role of the nurse from the role of the support worker. There was a fear that managers might fail to recognise this difference and see support workers as a cost-effective substitute for nurses.

It was also acknowledged that care giving sometimes relied on intuition. Nurses reported that the intuitive part of nursing was not always recognised and of feeling compromised when they verbalised their concerns.

> And if you tell them [the doctors] I'm worried or I'm concerned, or things just aren't right here, they kind of look at you. And if things kind of deteriorate, I feel kind of threatened when I ring them and say look you'd better get up here now. (G2, P2)

Clinical nurse specialists were considered a major resource in terms of their knowledge and expertise, especially when caring for patients with complex needs. However, they were also perceived as a threat. Concerns about the specialist role appeared to revolve around issues such as the risk of role erosion, with its associated undermining of the value of general nurses, and fragmentation of patient care. The need for greater harmony and understanding of each other's roles between ward staff and the clinical nurse specialists was recognised.

It was acknowledged that the future of the professional nurse was with the patient on an ongoing basis and that systems of care delivery such as primary nursing were the way forward. However, in reality nurses reported having to prioritise continually, the focus on task allocation with physical needs thus gaining priority. Being overwhelmed with work also had an impact on the nurses' aim to move the patient's health forward, as outlined by one respondent.

> Really what you're doing as a staff nurse is managing the morning or managing the afternoon and getting through that day. And it is difficult to stand back and see what those patients, with the patients obviously, what their care needs are. And how can you move them forward, because you're not concentrating on the whole picture. You're just concentrating on a very small part of it. (G4, P3)

Nurses acknowledged that task allocation militated against nurses exercising true responsibility and accountability for individualised patient care, but rather generated a collective diluted accountability and encouraged defensive practices.

Nurses also reported having little involvement in decision making at management level. Yet decisions made at this level were having a major impact on the nursing function and were sometimes leaving them open to litigation. This may be a further factor in encouraging defensive practices. It was suggested that defensive practices might also be due to educational deficits. In this respect, developments in nurse education were welcomed. Nurses also suggested that greater emphasis on nursing outcomes and on auditing nursing practices would serve to increase the value of the professional nurse and her contribution to patient care.

Pulling Everything Together

Pulling everything together is the term used to describe the coordinating role of the professional nurse. Nurses reported being responsible for the activities of various grades of staff and of being held to account when omissions or errors occurred, despite a perceived lack of autonomy to address problems.

The ward sister was reported to have a key role to play in maintaining morale among the multidisciplinary team. She was also considered pivotal to coordinating patient care activities and ensuring all necessary resources were available to effect a smooth delivery of service. However, all registered nurses reported that coordination was a significant aspect of their role.

> We call on the physiotherapist, we call on the dietician, we call on . . . the liaison nurse when they are going home. . . . If the rooms aren't being cleaned, we're looking after that, we're looking after the household and the staff. (G2, P3, 1, 2.)

Consequently, the extent of registered nurses' involvement in direct care giving appeared to be contingent upon the degree to which they were involved in coordinating ward activities. It also appeared to be influenced by the skill mix of staff available to give care. In wards with a favourable skill mix, most nurses reported a substantial contribution to direct care giving. However, on wards with a less favourable skill mix, as nurses had to supervise and check on the activities of more junior or unqualified staff, their contribution to direct patient care was proportionally lower.

With respect to nurse–doctor relationships, a complex picture emerges in the data. Nurses expressed the expectation that consultants would act as collegial and collaborative team members, while exercising account-ability for the smooth functioning of their own teams. Such a relationship appeared to exist in some situations. In others, however, a picture emerges of a lack of trust between nurses and doctors and, on occasions, the use of directive and bullying tactics by both groups. There was also an over-whelming perception that some junior doctors failed to pull their weight and did not receive adequate supervision from the more senior colleagues.

> We've begged for it. We even go down on the 1st of July and meet the interns and we encourage them and we say what our expectations are. And we give them a lot of time that first month. We've asked for follow up from SHOs and Registrars. We have never got it. (G1, P3)

As a consequence of this lack of support, the onus appeared to rest with nurses to check and supervise the work of junior doctors. Nurses reported being challenged by their own colleagues when interns failed to carry out duties assigned to them and also by consultants who appeared to hold nurses responsible. A cultural dependence by junior housemen on nursing staff was therefore fostered.

Thus pulling everything together describes another dimension of the nursing role. It was stated that trying to achieve a balance between giving care, supervising and coordinating was difficult and when the balance wasn't correct, patient outcomes were affected.

> There have been problems maybe when a student goes and does something wrong and maybe I haven't been able physically to be there to supervise and patients have ended up suffering. (G4, P1)

Nurses reported having to rely frequently on second-hand information regarding patient conditions. Meanwhile, reduced patient contact reflected on the amount of contextual information they were picking up. It was also noted that reduced involvement in patient care was undermining the patient's perception of the value of professional care giving. There was evidence of a reliance by patients on other grades to meet their needs and, indeed, of these grades doing a good job in this respect.

> Well, I had an experience this morning with one support worker. A patient who has been on the ward for quite a considerable amount of time said that this carer was his favourite nurse and I thought that spoke volumes about the support worker. Obviously, she was the person who was there with him most, taking him out for his little walks, taking him to the toilet, doing all those things in the past that nurses did and maybe what we still should be doing. (G4, P1).

The above scenario was leaving nurses feeling demoralised and undervalued.

Working Against the Odds to Move Nursing Forward

Working against the odds to move nursing forward is the core category which acts as a framework to integrate the three conceptual categories in order to describe the reality of being a general nurse.

Developing supportive–interactive relationships and knowledgeable care giving were integrally linked in that direct involvement in care giving facilitated the development of therapeutic relationships with patients, while a holistic knowledge of the patient served to inform and direct care giving. Coordinating the activities of the multidisciplinary team also served to inform nursing practice. Meanwhile, the closeness of the nurse–patient relationship put nurses in a unique position to advocate on behalf of patients with the multidisciplinary team. However, time spent supervising the activities of others was reducing nurses' contribution to direct care giving and thus interfering with their ability to sustain therapeutically effective relationships with patients. Fear of role erosion by clinical nurse specialists and support workers, who were picking up some of the deficits, was manifest. Operational policies were further fragmenting care, while perceived educational deficits were impacting on role articulation.

Overall a picture emerges of nurses being overwhelmed with work (role overload). In the process of trying to reconcile what the role of the nurses should be and what it appeared to entail, nurses were experiencing role conflict and ambiguity. It is possible that task allocation and its subsequent diluted accountability were used as a defence mechanism to offset the apparent stress nurses were experiencing. There was a realisation of the need for nurses to reprioritise their activities and become more integrally involved in patient care in order to move nursing forward. Further education to empower nurses and equip them with the necessary skills to provide an accountable service was also deemed necessary.

METHODOLOGICAL ISSUES

As already outlined, focus group interviews were used to collect data. All group participants indicated they had enjoyed the experience of being involved in a focus group interview and had found the interview process non-threatening. Consequently, it is possible that the interactive nature of focus group interviews yielded a more candid portrayal of reality than might have been obtained from individual interviews. Furthermore, discursive interaction frequently served to focus and clarify issues. Some nurses also felt that their participation in the focus group interviews had been a positive learning experience in that various problem-solving strategies used by others to resolve mutual difficulties were explored and evaluated.

Conversely, while the researcher found focus group interviews to be a very effective means of generating data, she encountered difficulties in ensuring a sufficient number of participants attended for interview. During the course of interviews, the researcher noted that there was invariably one participant in each group who was slow to become involved in discourse and who needed encouragement to express her views. Also, during the course of one focus group interview, the researcher had to intervene on a number of occasions to steer the conversation back to the topic of the research. Difficulties were further experienced in transcribing some of the data when all participants were talking simultaneously.

With respect to grounded theory methodology, the flexibility of this approach allowed for issues not previously considered by the researcher to be explored as they emerged. Furthermore, the rigorous analytic procedures involved in grounded theory served to offset the potential risk of premature closure or a subjective interpretation of data, which were both acknowledged risks as the researcher herself was a general nurse. However, while the researcher was at all times true to the data, dilemmas were encountered with respect to reporting on some issues which emerged. At the request of study participants, one short extract was removed from the findings section which, while true, participants felt might prove to be too contentious. Thus, it is possible that valuable data have been omitted which might have enriched the study findings.

The extent to which study findings reflect a national perspective on the role of the general nurse is questionable. The study was conducted in one study site only. It is also acknowledged that the sample population was devoid of any recently qualified staff. In retrospect, the researcher realised that the scope of the study was very broad. More in-depth information might have been obtained by narrowing the focus of the study. Consequently, findings of this pilot study are tentative and merit further empirical research.

CONCLUSION

The findings of this pilot study suggest that the role of the general nurse is currently moving along a continuum of change. While the reality of practice and its associated deficiencies are acknowledged, nurses appear to have a vision of what their role could and should entail. Meanwhile educational reforms, the introduction of clinical nurse specialists and support worker grades, while generally welcomed, serve to create uncertainty in some general nurses regarding the future of their roles. The divergence between nurses' aspirations to achieve their ideal role, role reality and future directions in the role of the nurse, is serving to create disharmony among the profession and a sense of disequilibrium.

Rheiner (1982) suggests that when disequilibrium occurs, unfavourable attitudes towards the institution frequently appear. The findings of this pilot study serve to confirm Rheiner's view. The perceived emphasis on cost-effectiveness, the reported lack of nursing involvement in decisions which are impacting on their practices, and a perception of role overload, are all deemed to diminish nurses' ability to provide a high quality nursing service. Meanwhile, on the one hand, the relative control that doctors still exercise over nursing practice and, on the other hand, their over reliance on nurses to inform their own practices are also seen to impede nursing development.

There are some correlations between the findings of this pilot study and the international literature, in which similar concerns are highlighted regarding the roles of support staff and clinical nurse specialists. The relative emphasis on cost containment is also reported. However, there appears to have been a greater degree of development of the professional role of the nurse outside Ireland. The findings of this pilot study suggest there is an emerging realisation that Irish nurses can redress some of their concerns themselves by reflecting on how care delivery actually occurs and implementing change to bring the professional nurse back to the bedside. This move should serve to create a greater valuing of the role of the professional nurse. Meanwhile, greater emphasis on developing relationships, based on trust and mutual respect, with the multidisciplinary team would serve to break down barriers. There is also a realisation that the future role of the general nurse is contingent upon their being appropriately educated so that they can proactively assume autonomous and accountable roles to give them the necessary resources to take nursing forward.

While the findings of this pilot study may appear to paint the view of a demoralised workforce and may be also somewhat contentious, it suggests that service managers need to re-evaluate seriously some of the policies which are currently interfering with the provision of a high quality nursing service. It also offers valuable insights into how the current uncertainty within the nursing profession can be redressed so as to optimise the contribution of Irish nurses within the health services.

RECOMMENDATIONS FOR FUTURE RESEARCH

This study appears to be the first study to explore the role of the general nurse as perceived and understood by a group of Irish general nurses. The extent to which the findings reflect the views of the body of Irish general nurses is unknown. It is recommended that further research is conducted to build on the findings of this pilot study so as to clarify and make explicit the role of the general nurse. With regard to nurses' use of intuition to inform their practices, there is a need for a comprehensive theoretical framework to describe intuition and therefore enhance its value. It is further recommended that research into nursing outcomes is undertaken in Ireland in order to validate the contribution of the professional nurse to the provision of a high quality service. The impact of educational reforms in Ireland on care provision also merits investigation, as does the impact of both support workers and clinical nurse specialists.

A number of issues arose in this pilot study regarding nurse-doctor relationships which have not been reported elsewhere. Further research on this topic among both nursing and medical cohorts might serve to clarify the dynamics of nurse-doctor interactions and how unequal power relationships could be redressed.

Although the Health Strategy (Department of Health, 1994) outlined three principles, including quality of care, which served to focus health service provision, the findings of this study suggest that cost considerations are the important criterion against which health services are currently being measured. It is recommended that health service managers utilise both qualitative and quantitative measures to evaluate outcomes and therefore achieve a more comprehensive picture of service delivery. With respect to costs and staffing determinants, it is essential that the Department of Health instigate national manpower studies to ensure that appropriate personnel, both in terms of skill and number, are available to provide a high quality nursing service to the public. The findings of this pilot study would indicate that current staffing levels are not appropriate to meet the needs of patients.

NOTE

1   In the study, a general nurse is defined as a professional nurse who is registered on the general division of the register maintained by An Bord Altranais, the Irish nursing registry and regulatory board.

REFERENCES

Albrecht, T.L., Johnson, G.M., and Walther, J.B. (1993) Understanding communication processes in focus groups, in: D Morgan (ed.), *Successful Focus Groups: Advancing the State of the Art*. London: Sage: 51–65.

Astedt-Kurki, P. and Haggman-Laitila, A. (1992) Good Nursing practice as perceived by clients: a starting point for the development of professional nursing, *Journal of Advanced Nursing,* 17 (10): 1195–9.

Ball, J.A., Hurst, K., Booth, M.R., and Franklin, R. (1989) *But Who Will Make the Beds?* Leeds: Mersey RHA and Nuffield Institute for Health Services Studies.

Basch, C. E. (1987) Focus Group Interview: an under-utilized research technique for improving theory and practice in health education, *Health Education Quarterly*, 14: 411–48.

Bousfield, C. (1997) A phenomenological investigation into the role of the clinical nurse specialist, *Journal of Advanced Nursing*, 25 (2): 245–56.

Bradshaw, P. (1996/1997) Going to Market: The effect of recent health reforms on the control and status of nursing work in British hospitals, *Nursing Review*, 15 (2): 66–9.

Carr-Hill, R., Dixon, P., Gibbs, I., Griffiths, M., Higgins, M., McCaughan, D., and Wright, K. (1992) *Skill Mix and the Effectiveness of Nursing Care*. University of York: Centre for Health Economics.

Chang, A.M. (1995) Perceived functions and usefulness of health service support workers, *Journal of Advanced Nursing*, 21 (1): 64–74

Commission on Nursing (1997) *Interim Report*. Dublin: Stationery Office.

Davies, S.M. (1992) Consequences of the division of nursing labour for elderly patients in continuing care settings, *Journal of Advanced Nursing*, 17 (5): 582–9.

Department of Health (1994) *Shaping a Healthier Future: A Strategy for Effective Healthcare in the 1990s*. Dublin: Stationery Office.

DHSS (Department of Health and Social Security) (1986) *Mix and Match: A Review of Nursing Skill Mix*. London: HMSO.

DHSS (Department of Health and Social Security) (1988) *Service Quality: A Report on the Activities of Nursing Staff on Hospital Wards: Report No 1/88*. NHS Management Consultancy Services/Nursing Division. London: HMSO.

Donovan M.I. and Lewis, G. (1987) Increasing productivity and decreasing costs: the value of RNs, *Journal of Nursing Administration*, 17 (9): 16–18.

Folch-Lyon, E. and Trost, J.F. (1981) Conducting Focus Group Sessions, *Studies in Family Planning*, 12 (12): 443–9.

Gavin, J. (1997) Nursing ideology and the 'generic carer', *Journal of Advanced Nursing*, 26 (4): 692–7.

Glaser, B.G. (1992) *Basics of Grounded Theory Analysis*. Mill Valley, CA: Sociology Press.

Glaser, B.G. and Strauss, A.L. (1967) *The discovery of Grounded Theory: Strategies for Qualitative Research*. Chicago: Aldine.

Guba, E.G. and Lincoln, Y.S. (1981) *Effective Evaluation: Improving the Usefulness of Evaluation Results through responses and Naturalist Approaches*. San Francisco: Jossey-Bass.

Hansler, D. and Cooper, C. (1986) Focus groups: new dimensions in feasibility study, *Fund Raising Management*, 12: 78–82.

Helt, E.H. and Jelinek, R.C. (1988) In the wake of cost cutting nursing productivity and quality improve, *Nursing Management*, 19 (6): 31–7.

Hicks, C. and Hennessy, D. (1998) Triangulation approach to the identification of acute sector nurses' training needs for formal nurse practitioner status, *Journal of Advanced Nursing*, 27 (1): 117–31.

Hinshaw, A.S., Scofield, R., and Atwood, J.R. (1981) Staff, patient and cost outcomes of all registered nurse staffing, *Journal of Nursing Administration*, 11: 30–6.

Kenney, J.W. (1995) Relevance of theory-based nursing practice, in: P.J. Christensen and J.W. Kenney (eds), *Nursing Process: Application of Conceptual Models* (4th edn). Missouri: Mosby: 3–23.

Kingry, M.J., Tiedje, L.B., and Friedman, L.L. (1990) Focus groups: a research technique for nursing, *Nursing Research*, 39 (2): 124–5.

Krueger, R.A. (1988) *Focus Groups: A Practical Guide for Applied Research*. California: Sage.

Lo-Biondo-Wood, G. and Haber, J. (1994) *Nursing Research Methods: Critical Appraisal and Utilization* (3rd edn). Missouri: Mosby.

McColl, E., Thomas, L., and Bond, S. (1996) A study to determine patient satisfaction with nursing care, *Nursing Standard*, 10 (52): 34–8.

Minyard, K., Wall, J., Turner, R. (1986) RNs may cost less than you think, *Journal of Nursing Administration*, 16 (5): 28–34.

Moores, B. and Thompson, A. (1986) What 1357 hospital inpatients think about aspects of their stay in British acute hospitals, *Journal of Advanced Nursing*, 11 (1): 87–102.

Morgan, D. (1992) Designing focus group research, in: M. Steward, F. Tudiver, M. Bass, E. Dunn, P. Norton (eds), *Tools for Primary Care Research*. California: Sage: 177–193.

Morse, J.M. (1995) *Qualitative Nursing Research: A Contemporary Dialogue*. California: Sage.

Nyamathi, A. and Shuler, P. (1990) Focus group interview: a research technique for informed nursing practice, *Journal of Advanced Nursing*, 15 (11): 1281–8.

Pearson, A., Punton, S., and Durant, L. (1987) *Nursing Beds: An Evaluation of the Effects of Therapeutic Nursing*. Harrow: Scutari Press.

Rheiner, N.W. (1982) Role theory: framework for change, *Nursing Management*, 13: 20–2.

Richardson, G. and Maynard, A. (1995) *Fewer Doctors? More Nurses? A Review of the Knowledge Base of Doctor-Nurse Substitution*, Discussion Paper 135. University of York: Centre for Health Economics.

Royal College of Nursing (RCN) (1992) *The Value of Nursing*. London: Royal College of Nursing.

Sandelowski, M. (1986) The problem of rigour in qualitative research, *Advances in Nursing Science*, 8 (3): 27–37.

Savage, E. (1997) Paranursing: Establishing the boundaries, *The World of Irish Nursing*, 5 (6): 18–19.

Strauss, A. and Corbin, J. (1990) *Basics of Qualitative Research: Grounded Theory Procedures and Techniques*. London: Sage.

Thornley, C. (1997) *The Invisible Workers: An Investigation into the Pay and Employment of HCAs*. London: Unison.

Weston, D., Bruster, S., Lorentzon, M., and Bosanquet, N. (1995) The management of quality assurance in nursing, *Journal of Nursing Management*, 3 (5): 229–36.

White, R. (1988). The influence of nursing on the politics of health, in: R. White (ed.), *Political Issues in Nursing: Past, Present and Future* (Vol. 3). New York: John Wiley: 15–31.

12

Hospital Nurses' Perceptions of Health Promotion

Margaret P. Treacy and Rita Collins

INTRODUCTION

This chapter reports on research that was carried out between 1995 and 1996.[1] It presents part of the findings from that study, which describe hospital nurses' understanding, involvement in and perspectives on health promotion. It is suggested that nursing, midwifery and health professions can play a dominant role in health promotion (Mahler, 1985; Parish, 1987; King, 1994; Department of Health, 1994; Department of Health, 1995). However, the term 'health promotion', while gaining widespread usage and popularity in recent years, has a wide range of meanings (Schultz, 1991; Latter et al., 1992; Tones, 1993; Dines and Cribb, 1993; Delaney, 1994). Duncan and Gold (1986) suggest that it has become 'an all inclusive umbrella term'. Few Irish studies exploring nurses' involvement in or attitudes to health promotion have been undertaken (apart from Burke, 1986; Treacy, 1987; O'Sullivan, 1995).

Prior to the Ottawa Charter (WHO, 1986), attempts to promote health were referred to as health education. Conventional health education focused on the giving of information and attempting to modify individuals' attitudes and behaviours (Naidoo and Wills, 1994; Ewles and Simnett, 1995). Health promotion is broader than this (Caraher, 1994a), aiming to protect or improve health by focusing on behavioural, socio-economic and environmental changes (Catford and Nutbeam, 1984). A common misconception which emerges in the literature is the interchangeable use of the term health education and health promotion, although distinctions have been outlined (Stachtchenko and Jenicek, 1990).

Many writers attest to the fact that nurses have a role to play in health promotion (Melvin, 1987; Soeken et al., 1989; Donoghue et al., 1990; Latter et al., 1992; Gorin, 1992; Delaney, 1994; King, 1994). Health promotion and health education are therefore deemed to be a central element of the nurse's role. Reasons provided for this assertion include the fact that nurses are deemed to occupy a position of close continuous contact with clients and are a large occupational group within the health services. In quantitative studies both McBride (1994) and Mitchinson (1995) found that the majority of nurses perceived that they had a role to play in health promotion. However it is suggested that for nurses to be effective in health promotion or health education educational change is nesessary (Macleod Clark and Webb, 1985). In addition Macleod Clark (1993) notes that if nurses are to realise an effective role in health promotion it is essential that a reappraisal of relationships between nurses and patients takes place.

A central misconception surrounding nurses' perception of health promotion is the equation of health promotion with health education, which can lead to a very narrow understanding of health promotion. Gott and O'Brien (1990a) argue that definitions of health promotion within nursing, and trends within nursing in general, promote an individualistic approach to the promotion of health. In a qualitative study of a mixed group of registered nurses they found that on the one hand nurses distinguished nursing from health promotion, feeling that nursing was the 'hands on' delivery of care. On the other hand they put nursing and health promotion together and argued that nurses were 'facilitators towards health' (Gott and O'Brien, 1990a). Nurses tended to view health promotion as the transmission of information and did not appear to have internalised ideas about client participation in care. Another qualitative study of ward sisters and charge nurses found that ward sisters viewed health promotion and health education as one and the same (Latter, 1993). Non research-based work also maintains that in health promotion where responsibility for health is placed on the individual, nurses adopt a 'victim blaming' approach (Caraher, 1994b), and Delaney (1994) states that nursing has viewed health promotion in terms of 'individual disease prevention' and failed to take account of cultural and economic factors. However, Davis (1995) in a qualitative study explored rehabilitation nurses' understanding of and role in health education and health promotion, and found that respondents identified the same aim in both health promotion and rehabilitation nursing, namely, encouraging clients to manage their own care. Both Caraher (1994a) and Gott and O'Brien (1990b), who employed the broader concept of health promotion as outlined in the Ottawa Charter (WHO, 1986), suggest that nurses carry out little health promotion.

The Practice of Health Promotion in Nursing

A survey aimed at examining the health education role and practices of nurses in acute care areas indicates that nurses operate within the traditional medical model of health retaining the balance of power in client–nurse interactions (Latter et al., 1992). Caraher (1994a) makes similar claims which are also supported by the work of Gott and O'Brien (1990a) who found that nurses adopt an authoritative guidance approach when undertaking health promotion activities. The process and outcome of nurses' interventions in relation to smoking cessation was explored by Macleod Clark et al. (1990). They found that in 58 per cent of recordings nurses talked considerably more than clients and generally controlled the conversations. In addition the tapes revealed that nurses tended to resort to prescriptive advice, telling patients what was 'best' for them to do rather than allowing them to make their own choices and decisions. Advice giving appears to be the predominant health promotion activity of participants in their study.

While nurses appear to value health promotion the extent of their activities in this area has been shown to be limited. When asked why they failed to give advice to clients, nurses identified time constraints, lack of training (McBride, 1994; Mitchinson, 1995), and the absence of a structured approach to recording nursing interventions (McBride, 1994). Gott and O'Brien (1990b) suggest that nurses do not carry out health promotion activities as outlined in the Ottawa Charter (WHO, 1986) and require education rather than training for this role. They state that nurses do not possess all the necessary knowledge and skills to fulfil the health promotion role that could be expected of them. Gott and O'Brien (1990b) also question the holistic and consequently individualistic aspect of nursing models. Treacy (1987) in an Irish study on nursing and health education suggests that as nurses are disempowered within the hospital setting they are unable to take on a role which empowers others. Both Tones (1993) and Macleod Clark (1993) note that health promotion can occur only in the context of empowerment and partnership. At another level, Caraher (1994a) suggests that the hospital structure, in which patient compliance is required to ensure the smooth running of the service, discourages client autonomy and militates against health promotion.

Quantitative studies (Latter et al., 1992; McBride, 1994; Mitchinson, 1995) indicate that nurses consider they have a role to play in health promotion. This work also indicates that nurses adopt top-down approaches and focus on individual lifestyle advice. However, these studies by virtue of their design have not fully explored nurses' perceptions of the concept of health promotion. Any development of a health promotion role for nurses must be based on an individual's understanding of the concept.

The qualitative studies (Treacy, 1987; Gott and O'Brien, 1990a; Davis, 1995; Latter, 1993) discussed are limited by virtue of the group/groups studied, nevertheless they provide an understanding of how the nurses included in the studies perceive health promotion. This chapter presents the results of similar exploratory work undertaken with registered nurses in Ireland.

RESEARCH AIMS AND STRATEGY

This study focused on exploring hospital nurses' understanding of health promotion and their perceptions of their nursing practice in relation to health promotion activities.[2] A qualitative methodology was used given that it was important to explore nurses' understanding and experiences from their own perspective and to avoid imposing preconceived meanings and assumptions.[3] Grounded theory was selected as the approach to this study. The purpose of grounded theory is to build theory from the data collected (Strauss and Corbin, 1990). This technique was developed by Glaser and Strauss (1967) and it allows exploration of reality as experienced by the individual. The main data collection method used in the study was the depth interview. A topic guide was used to help focus the interview, while allowing the individual perspectives and experiences of participants to emerge. Depth interviewing allows the interviewees to respond and express their own perspective in their own words and allows the researcher to hear what is in the mind of another (Patton, 1980).

The Sample

Registered nurses included in the study were selected from four large teaching hospitals, two within Dublin and two outside Dublin. Hospitals were chosen on the basis that they served wide catchment areas and provided care for clients of differing age, sex and socio-economic status. This allowed for differences in the way nurses might experience health promotion in different settings to be explored.

All participants were in full-time employment in the hospital setting, were registered general nurses qualified for a minimum of two years and all were working in acute general care settings but not in coronary care or intensive care.[4]

Participant selection within the hospitals adopted a random format. One registered nurse who fulfilled the inclusion criteria was randomly selected from each non-specialist ward in all of the four hospitals and asked to participate in the study. In total, 47 hospital-based registered general nurses participated in the study.

Ethical Issues

Institutions included in the study were initially approached for permission to undertake the research and to contact nurses working in potential study units. Information regarding the study was given to potential participants and it was stressed that participation was voluntary. Individual verbal agreement to participate was sought from all participants. Interviews were timetabled at a future date after the initial consent was given by the individual concerned. This allowed participants further opportunity for reflection on their participation. Consent was obtained by the interviewer in all cases. Participants were assured of anonymity and confidentiality.

The Interview[5]

All of the interviews were carried out by one interviewer and were tape-recorded and transcribed verbatim. Respondents were informed that the interviewer had a nursing background. It was felt that while this could introduce an element of bias, on balance it would enhance the quality of the data generated. Respondents could develop a better rapport with a nurse and they might be more open and willing to discuss their practices.

Data Analysis

Data analysis follows Strauss's and Corbin's (1990) approach of open, axial and selective coding and is informed by other work (Glaser and Strauss, 1967; Strauss and Corbin, 1990; Sarantakos, 1994). Data were broken down initially and conceptualised, then clusters of data which appeared to fit together were grouped while identifying similarities and differences. Using the constant comparative method, categories were developed and described. A number of categories were identified in this study and data were not compressed into a single core category.

Methodological Issues

A variety of suggestions appear in the literature with regard to the establishment of rigour in qualitative research. In order to assess grounded theory research it is proposed that the research process must be made explicit so that judgments can be made regarding 'fit with reality', provision of understanding, and utility (Strauss and Corbin, 1990). Burnard (1991) suggests that there are two ways of establishing validity in qualitative research – member and expert checks. Lincoln and Guba (1985) suggest four criteria for establishing rigour: 'truth value', 'applicability', 'consistency' and 'neutrality'. There is some overlap between these criteria; Sandelowski (1986) describes them as follows. Truth value has to do with the researcher accurately seeing and representing phenomena being studied from the perspective of participants. Truth value is judged in terms of credibility which relates to 'faithful description' of participants' experiences. Ways of ensuring faithful description include audio/video taping participants' accounts (Sandelowski, 1998), 'member checking' or asking study participants to check accuracy of interview accounts. Faithful description can also be reflected when others identify the experience from the description given in the research report. Applicability is judged in terms of 'fittingness'. Fittingness is comprised of three aspects: applicability of findings beyond the study setting; when others can relate findings to their own similar situation, and when the data reported support the interpretation presented. Consistency is judged in terms of 'auditability' and this is demonstrated when the decision trail is presented clearly so that other researchers can potentially arrive at similar conclusions. Neutrality, in terms of confirmability, is attained when truth value, applicability and consistency are demonstrated (Sandelowski, 1986).

Sandelowski (1998) indicates that both member and expert checks can be problematic in qualitative research and that the onus is always on the researcher to demonstrate the grounds for interpretation. Member checks were not a feature of this study but interviews were tape-recorded and transcribed verbatim to ensure accuracy of data. Colleagues informally acted as 'expert sounding boards' at various stages of the study but were not asked to validate category generation. Sandelowski (1998) suggests that outside experts do not have the immersion in data to undertake this task which must rest with the researcher. In qualitative research it is suggested that validity is the result of researcher integrity. This is an emerging issue in qualitative research which has to be addressed. Issues of bias in this study could arise in relation to interviews which were all conducted by a nurse interviewer; as indicated this could have precluded discussion with an immersion in 'taken for granted' understanding of nursing practices. On balance, however, it is felt that this fact added to the quality of data generated. As with qualitative work a judgement sample was used. No claims are made for the applicability of findings beyond the study setting; it is anticipated, however, that registered nurses can relate to aspects of the experiences described. Category saturation was reached and categories presented represent a plausible interpretation of the experiences of the nurses studied. In this report verbatim extracts from interviews are presented together with interpretation so that readers can make their own assessment of this aspect of fittingness. The various stages of the research process are clearly outlined in the study thus highlighting the decision trail. However, it must be acknowledged that there are multiple interpretations along with multiple experiences of reality (Sandelowski, 1993). What this report presents is an interpretation which is grounded in the data.

FINDINGS

Findings from the study, addressing participants' understanding and perception of health promotion and their engagement therein, are presented as two categories each comprising a number of properties or themes. The two categories address participants' perceptions of health promotion and health education, and practices in relation to health promotion.

Perceptions of Health Promotion and Health Education

This category is made up of three sub-categories and describes participants' understanding of the concepts of health promotion and health education. It suggests an uncertainty regarding the concept of health promotion and identifies a lack of shared understanding of the concept among participants.

Health promotion and health education – 'I'm not sure'
This sub-category indicates that nurses have difficulty in defining both health promotion and health education.

> . . . cause I'm amazed . . . , you know, I can't even explain to you what health education is or health promotion is. (P26)

When pressed participants gave common-sense rather than professional definitions of health education and health promotion. They struggled to define both concepts and could only do so by defining the words 'promotion' and 'education'.

> . . . Health education you are educating people, promotion you might try to promote a product or promote something, education you are actually . . . teaching someone how to be healthy or they should do this or that where promoting people might be telling people directly what they should do.(P34)

Because health promotion was defined by participants as concerned with 'educating the public', it followed that health promotion occurred in the community or outside the hospital.

> [Health promotion is] . . . improving existing standards and increasing awareness and knowledge for people in the community as opposed to in-hospital situations. (P12)

In general nurses linked health promotion to public campaigns and to television or poster advertisements.

Health promotion is 'broad', health education has a 'specific purpose'
In this sub-category, health promotion was described by participants as 'broad' whereas health education was considered to have a specific goal or specific intended outcome.

> [health education] . . . you're educating on a specific purpose, you've a certain goal at the end of it and health promotion I suppose is just a more broad-based thing (P21)

> . . . the health education week that you hear about, has a more definite, it strikes home more, because there is more people behind it and maybe have more backup. Whereas I found with health promotion, a lot of the time it is just leaflets that I see around the place. (P15)

In some sense participants perceived health education to have a specific goal and they indicated that it could occur within the hospital or health sector.

'Health promotion and health education are the same'
Most participants also thought health promotion and health education went together and that there was little or no difference between the two.

> Health promotion and health education are the same really. Promoting good health again in a patient, is the same as educating them as a nurse. I would have thought they are both the same. (P7)

> They're kinda similar aren't they? (P31)

This sub-category highlights participants' lack of clarity regarding the concept.

The category indicates that participants were not sure about health promotion or health education. The varying interpretations they offered were sometimes at variance with previous statements. Participants did not discuss partnership with or the empowerment of patients.

It was suggested that health promotion was concerned with 'educating the public about health' and chiefly occurred outside the hospital or health sector, and health education was concerned with 'teaching about health'. Generally participants thought that there was a difference but they had difficulty in articulating it. Accounts suggest that nurses do not fully understand the concepts as reflected in the dominant literature and are not operating from a shared understanding of health promotion or health education.

Nurses' Practices in Relation to Health Promotion

Participants' attitudes to and involvement in what they see as health promotion activities in their day-to-day work are described in the five sub-categories which comprise this category. It is interesting to note that, despite their difficulty in articulating the meaning of health promotion, participants had little difficulty discussing their health promotion role. The category indicates the types of health promotion activities which participants consider are part of their role.

Giving advice

Participants perceive their role as health promoters to be that of 'giving advice'. Participants indicated that they could give patients 'basic' advice but needed to refer patients to specialists for more in-depth advice.[6] They stated that health promotion could be located in the patient teaching aspect of their role. When asked if health promotion is recognised as a nursing activity a nurse replies:

> Not on those terms, but we would call it teaching a patient. That would be recognised as a nursing activity. (P3)

A minority of participants believed that they had a role to play in advising patients about general health issues, in addition to informing them about their specific complaint.

> They've come into hospital and had an illness and they've had a condition wrong with them or whatever . . . in order for them to prevent that happening again, you have to teach them about it and what they can do to prevent that and encourage them to take the right line of approach and adapting their lifestyle. (P8)

The type of information given by participants tended to be specific to the condition with which the patient had been admitted.

> . . . like people who have gall bladder problem, you know, their diet is very important, they have to have a certain diet, low fat, and . . . diabetics, as well, . . . these type of people need education on a regular basis. (P37)

Accounts suggest that once they have advised patients, participants considered their intervention to be complete. Some uncertainty was expressed regarding a patient education role for nurses.

> . . . a lot of time, we don't know if we are supposed to do these things or not. Whether it is part of your job or not, to do health promotion or even to tell people. (P15)

Despite some doubts most participants believe that they should educate clients and that the health promotion aspect of their role is reflected in 'advice giving' to patients.

'It's just part of our normal routine'
Participants viewed health promotion, as in advice giving, as an integral part of their daily routine delivery of nursing care.

> . . . we are doing health promotion every day but we don't realise it, it is just part of our normal routine. One example is mobilising . . . We mobilise patients every day and it is just kind of routine you know . . . just giving them drinks, you are still promoting health you know. (P17)

In general nurses felt that, as they assisted patients towards a return to their normal 'healthy' role, they engaged in health promotion. This taken for granted aspect of their health promotion role is also opportunistic and unplanned. The following describes when health promotion occurs:

> In the course of our work we don't set out with a plan . . . doing the beds in the morning, bathing someone. (P9)

However, the onus of initiating discussion is often left to the patient; unsolicited information is not given.

> I think more often than not they ask us. I am under the impression that we should be doing it more. You're offering advice to them rather than waiting for them to ask. (P1)

Where health promotion occurred, and when it was not patient initiated, it was often prompted by two events, the patient's admission or discharge. On admission nurses identify patients' problems or potential problems.

> . . . when they [patients] are admitted first, they [nurses] go over this list of activities of daily living so you would be going through a lot of their lifestyle there like whether they are mobile and whether they smoke, whether they . . . a lot of physiological things and physical things that they might need help with, mobilising, sleeping and eating and all those things so you could assess them quite a good bit there on admission as well. (P42)

Discharge was the last occasion on which nurses would see the patient and therefore presented the last opportunity to give advice.

> Specifically when they are going home you make time to talk to them, go through their tablets, make sure of their appointment for coming back and going through all those things with them. (P16)

Information given to patients by nurses is arbitrary and is generally concerned with passing on information relating to the patient's immediate concerns. It is often intended to keep them going until their next appointment as an outpatient.

This sub-category demonstrates that participants consider that they undertake health promotion on a daily basis as a routine part of their job. They suggest that it occurs in a general way as they assist patients towards recovery and in specific 'advice giving' aspects of their role. However, it is unplanned and is carried out only if the opportunity arises. It is sometimes dependent on the patient initiating the encounter by asking questions.

'It's not a priority'

This sub-category describes how health promotion features in the daily work routine of participants. It also implicitly describes barriers to health promotion. Participants indicate that health promotion, which they define as 'giving advice', is carried out only after all other work is completed and the patient's physical needs are met. Participants attributed this to the need to get through the ward workload that is geared to the immediate physical needs of patients.

> If you . . . take time to sit down and talk to a patient, some people might be thinking 'well I've all these other things to be doing' . . . and if their seniors don't approve of what they're doing, I mean, if they're getting negative feedback from there . . . (P26)

Getting through the work dominated the participants' day to such an extent that they perceived they had not the time to explain to patients what they were doing. Health promotion in the form of patient education was an 'optional' extra and the least important aspect of that workload.

> . . . it is just as important to give that man the answers he needs to all his questions and educate him regarding certain aspects of his care, as to dress his wound. In my opinion the nursing care comes first, his wound, his general day to day care but it is just as important to educate that man. (P2)

The relatively low priority of health promotion is indicated by the fact that the health promotion activities of nurses are rarely or inadequately documented.

> You tend to document more what is going to be a treatment than what is education. You don't document really anything that you might have spent time talking about their illness. You just don't document that, you document things that are actually procedures not what you are actually saying to patients. (P34)

Where it is documented, no account is given of goals set or information given; only general global statements are recorded. Participants indicated that nurses communicate verbally with their colleagues about health promotion activities and what actions they have taken, but it is not planned or documented. They indicated that when health promotion activities were documented it was often for legal reasons, for example when a patient ignores advice.

To summarise, this sub-category demonstrated that health promotion activities were very much subordinate to meeting patients' physical needs. There is a sense in which because it is not 'doing' that it is not real work. Thus health promotion is fitted in when time permits. Participants believed that health promotion might not be valued by their nursing colleagues. The fact that health promotion activities are not documented means that such aspects of care, namely advice, information giving or psychological support become 'invisible', unacknowledged and unrewarded aspects of nurses' work. It also means that nurses lack role models in relation to this activity.

'We refer patients'
Participants described ensuring that patients are referred to the appropriate specialist as an important aspect of their role as health promoters. This sub-category 'we refer patients' suggests that nurses play the role of coordinator and ensure patients are referred to the appropriate healthcare specialist or clinical nurse specialist. Participants state that they also mediate on the patient's behalf by identifying a problem or potential problem and referring the patient to the appropriate specialist.

> . . . really it boils down to the nurse to try and get these other various professionals to the ward to see these people, you know, to give them their specialised care if that's what's needed and to let them get on with it. (P66)

Participants considered that their function was to reinforce the specialist's advice.

> Inhaler technique and everything, the asthma nurse would come up and show the patients how to do it and then she'll let us know how well she thinks they're doing so you just have to really reiterate what she has said to them. (P22)

It was indicated that clinical nurse specialists were more knowledgeable and therefore were better able to educate patients.

> . . . They [specialist nurses] have all the information at hand which an ordinary staff nurse on a ward wouldn't have just at their fingertips. (P36)

The presence of clinical nurse specialists or other specialists resulted in some respondents believing that they had no role to play in educating patients. Others made the point that they knew as much as specialist nurses but did not have the time to teach patients.

Because they [specialist nurses] have the time, that is the biggest thing, in their chosen fields they have the expertise . . . , because they have the time to sit and talk . . . (P3)

Clinical nurse specialists were considered by most participants to be better able to educate patients because they have the time, more up-to-date knowledge and patient contact. Participants ensure patients are referred to the appropriate specialist or clinical nurse specialist. It gives nurses one less job to do and they reinforce the specialists' input. This sub-category describes a coordinating or mediating role.

'You keep trying'

This sub-category suggests that participants had an interest in health promotion as reflected in advice and information giving activities. Accounts suggest that participants persist in these activities in the absence of results or feedback.

You wonder is it worth trying again, obviously, but I don't think you give up. . . . you mightn't be as strong about it or, you know, be as forceful, if forceful is the right word but you don't give up because you know that is your role and you are doing it for the best. (P43)

Participants indicated that in their experience if they explained to the patient about their condition it helped the patients' recovery, reduced their anxiety and enabled them to play an active role in their care.

Even when somebody comes in, prior to surgery, . . . the difference in the person, after things have been explained . . . the calmness that comes over them is unbelievable, when things are explained properly. (P15)

Participants were unsure, however, whether all of the health promotion activities they carried out were effective, principally because they frequently did not see the outcome of their intervention.

You never know if it's goin' to be a hundred per cent effective because a lot of people go out and possibly you aren't goin' to see them again . . . (P22)

In this sub-category participants indicated that it was important to keep up health promotion activities in terms of giving advice even in the absence of positive outcomes. Participants appeared to be 'interested' in health promotion because it either helped to prevent illness or helped patients to cope with their condition. However, participants received limited feedback and were unsure if the health promotion they carried out was effective.

SUMMARY

In this category participants described their health promotion role as the provision of information for patients. Advice given by nurses appeared to be standardised, prescriptive and specific to the patient's condition. Accounts suggest that nurses viewed advice giving as an integral part of their role and that their health promotion activities tended to be somewhat ad hoc. Accounts also suggest that for nurses health promotion activities are not of primary concern and that getting through the work, and caring for patients' physical needs take precedence. In addition and not unrelated is the issue that health promotion activities by nurses are rarely or poorly documented. Participants view themselves as coordinators of patients' care. They believe their role is to reinforce the advice given to the patient by healthcare specialists and particularly clinical nurse specialists. Participants continue to advise patients even if they appear to be unresponsive. However, they received only limited feedback on the effectiveness of their interventions. Accounts make it clear that when participants talked about their role in health promotion they were discussing a very limited patient teaching role with short-term goals of getting the patient through their hospitalisation period.

DISCUSSION

Almost all registered nurses in this qualitative study felt they should be engaged in health promotion activities in terms of health teaching and the promotion of health. Other research reports similar findings (McBride, 1994; Mitchinson, 1995). Participants in this study were at variance with dominant views of health promotion and health education as reflected in the literature. They were unable to distinguish between health promotion, health education and general information giving. This is not a new issue in nursing but it is one which has to be borne in mind when considering the potential nurses have as health promoters. A similar lack of understanding of health promotion by nurses is also reflected in UK literature (Gott and O'Brien, 1990a; Delaney, 1994; Maben and Macleod Clark, 1995). A more recent study found that newly qualified diplomats discussed dominant views of health education/health promotion (Macleod Clark and Maben, 1998). However when this was explored in terms of their practice the diplomats had a more traditional perspective and viewed health promotion and health education as an activity involving individual teaching related to lifestyle and behaviour change.

In this study participants did not identify a preventive dimension to their role and tended to consider health promotion activities as something that 'happened in the community'. This indicates that hospital nurses operate within a very narrow curative model, which acts as a barrier to their health promotion role. Melvin (1987) suggests that health visitors have a more visible health promotion role than other nurses and Caraher (1994b) also notes that nurses outside the hospital setting are more closely associated with health promotion.

The category describing 'nurses' practices in relation to health promotion' indicates that the awareness of health promotion as an important aspect of nursing care was not actually realised in practice. The students included in Macleod Clarke's and Maben's (1998) study also perceived health education/health promotion in terms of individual teaching and behaviour change. In this study only one registered nurse spoke of the optimal health of an individual when discussing health promotion although some had a sense that is was 'broader' than health education. Where participants described what they considered to be health promotion, it tended to be in relation to what is described as patient education in the nursing literature (Tones et al., 1990). Patient education is related to the patient's presenting condition whereas health education has a more general focus (Tones, et al., 1990). Nursing tends to view health promotion as individual disease prevention (Gott and O'Brien, 1990a; Delaney, 1994). Caraher (1998) attempts to analyse the relationship between patient education and health promotion and discusses clinical health promotion as a more useful term to describe a health promotion role for hospital nurses. Clinical health promotion encompasses the process of patient education but requires a new approach to patients by health professionals; it is 'concerned with relationships and partnership arrangements' (Caraher, 1998: 57).

A feature of nursing practice which impacts on health promotion is the idea that 'talking isn't working' (Melia, 1987; Treacy, 1987). Accounts in this study incorporate similar beliefs as participants report the need to get on with the physical work of 'doing' in nursing. Health promotion, which may involve talking without 'doing', is not a priority. Accounts indicate that nurses rarely take time out of their routine work to talk to patients. When they do, it is usually in relation to giving condition-related information during hospitalisation or on discharge. Participants do not normally engage in a form of patient teaching which is an overt aspect of their work.

Participants' accounts of their role in advice giving to clients give little indication of a partnership approach. Accounts suggest that they tend to carry out patient teaching, or, as they see it, health promotion, in a prescriptive manner. They focus on the individual rather than taking account of the wider, social, political and environmental issues. The approach does not incorporate the advocacy, empowerment and mediation aspects of the Ottawa Charter (WHO, 1986). A prescriptive approach by nurses to giving health advice and information and a failure to recognise the client's perspective or to encourage client participation has been noted by others (Gott and O'Brien, 1990a; Macleod Clark et al., 1990). The question must be asked if the traditional culture of nursing or the culture of the modern hospital supports a preventive role by nurses. Robinson and Hill (1995) note the complexity of changes required if Project 2000 nurses are to become health promoters. While Piper and Browne (1998) note the complexity of nurses engagement in empowering activities with clients.

A minority of participants in this study felt they should not give advice to patients. In McBride's (1994) study, a minority (15.7 per cent) of respondents also felt they should not give health promotion advice. This indicates a confusion that exists for some nurses in relation to their role. Most participants felt that they could undertake the job of patient teaching if they had the time. However many felt that health promotion activities, that is patient education in relation to particular conditions, were increasingly the domain of clinical nurse specialists because they considered them to have greater expertise. The general phenomenon of referring patients to others is also reflected in other work (McBride, 1994).

Accounts indicate that health promotion activities were generally unplanned and undocumented. This makes these aspects of nursing workload invisible and perhaps less valued by nurses and their colleagues. The failure to record health promotion interventions has also been noted elsewhere and identified as a barrier to health promotion activities by nurses (McBride, 1994). Macleod Clark (1993) notes that research findings indicate that interventions for smoking cessation which succeed are distinguished by clear indicators of the nurse's intervention style. This failure to plan and/or record aspects of nursing care is a general issue in nursing. Developments such as the introduction of the nursing process (Basford and Slevin, 1995) may assist in refocusing and establishing an overt approach to the patient education aspects of nursing, although Gott and O'Brien (1990b) warn against the individualistic approach of many nursing models.

In describing their role as health promoters, hospital-based nurses indicate that they 'keep trying' and that they see value in health promotion, in their terms health teaching related to patients' presenting condition and immediate needs. Apart from reduction of patient anxiety by information giving, participants were unable to comment on the effectiveness of their activities in effecting lifestyle behaviour change. They attributed this to the short length of patient stay and their inability to follow up patients. It is also related to lack of planning and documentation. This may contribute to a lack of interest in health promotion on the part of some respondents. Literature from the UK gives mixed responses on nurses' perceived effectiveness of health promotion. McBride's (1994) study indicates disagreement among nurse participants regarding their ability to change lifestyle behaviour while Vincent et al. (1985) and Holcomb and Mullen (1986) found a degree of pessimism among nurses regarding behaviour change.

Macleod Clark (1993) states that the principles which support nursing practice must enhance health. She suggests that a professional revolution is required in order to shift away from sick nursing to a health nursing model. In the UK it was found that traditional approaches which emphasised physical health were predominant, and although health promotion and health were included in the curriculum, they featured in an irregular and piecemeal fashion (Lask et al., 1994). Nurse education programmes in the UK, despite attempts at refocusing curricula to incorporate health promotion still retain deficiencies in this respect (Lask et al., 1994). The Syllabus for General Nurse Training (An Bord Altranais, 1993) simply lists health education with sub-headings of mental health and physical health.[7] In acknowledging the importance of focusing Irish nurse education to incorporate preparation for primary health care roles, it is suggested that student nurses should have more community nursing experience in their training (An Bord Altranais, 1994; Department of Health, 1994). Changes also include additional input on social and behavioural sciences, which may help nurses to contextualise their care and provide them with a broader framework within which to locate their nursing interventions. However, changes recently introduced, and currently being proposed, in nurse education in Ireland do not necessarily include a refocusing of the curriculum towards health or health promotion. The way in which the ethos of health promotion (advocacy, empowerment and mediation) is represented to nurses in training has to be considered.

Many of the proposals for change in the UK where similar difficulties have been identified centre on 'individual' change, that is, refocusing the education and training of the nurse. While findings from this study support these proposals, Gott and O'Brien (1990c) point out that the status and authority of nurses – the conditions for full participation in bringing about structural changes which impact on health – are not present. In another study it is suggested that nurses are disempowered and hence cannot participate fully in health education (Treacy, 1987). In analysing health promotion Tones (1993) suggests that empowerment is the main function of health education and that nurses need to be empowered themselves so that they can empower patients.

This study has identified a number of issues to consider if nurses are to realise their potential as health promoters. It raises questions about participants' preparation for a health promotion role and aspects of current approaches to nursing care, which may militate against such a role.

Findings identify a lack of clarity regarding the concept of health promotion, and work practices and a work environment which does not value health promotion activities. These findings provide direction for bringing about change. However, prior to identifying interventions based on this qualitative study, it is important that the generalisability of these findings be established with a representative sample of registered general nurses.

ACKNOWLEDGEMENTS

The authors gratefully acknowledge the contribution to the report on which this paper is based of Dympna Casey, who acted as research assistant for a major part of this project and Adeline Cooney, who provided invaluable assistance in the course of the study. A special thank you is also extended to the nurses who participated in this study. The project was funded by the Department of Health.

NOTES

1 Only part of the data set is presented here. Other data sets will be published elsewhere. This research was funded by the Department of Health and was part of a study carried out to explore the attitudes of nurses to their own health and personal lifestyle habits, and to their health promotion activities in relation to coronary heart disease (Treacy et al., 1996).

2 The research on which this chapter is based included both hospital and public health nurses. This chapter presents and discusses findings in relation to hospital-based nurses.

3 In addition nurses also completed a questionnaire dealing with health life practices and their knowledge of cardiovascular disease prevention. These findings are presented elsewhere (Treacy et al., 1996).

4 It was considered that interviewing nurses qualified for more than two years would provide a more reflective or mature account of what actually took place in nursing practice in terms of health promotion. Including specialist nurses in the study could distort findings and it was decided to concentrate on the non-specialist general registered nurses' perceptions and experiences in relation to health promotion. All participants were engaged in the care of adult patients.

5 Initial interviews were developmental and assessed the scope and value of the interview schedule and gave some indication of the time required for interviews.

6 The reasons why respondents needed to refer patients are described in greater detail within the theme 'we refer patients'.

7 Although individual curricula in schools of nursing may incorporate elements of health promotion teaching, this content has yet to be evaluated in current curricula. A new syllabus for general nursing training is in the process of being developed.

204 *Nursing Research: Design and Practice*

REFERENCES

Basford, L. and Slevin, O. (1995) *Theory and Practice of Nursing.* Edinburgh: Campion Press.

An Bord Altranais (1994) *The Future of Nurse Education and Training in Ireland.* Dublin: An Bord Altranais.

An Bord Altranais (1993) *Syllabus for the Education and Training of Student Nurses (general).* Dublin: An Bord Altranais.

Burke, T. P. (1986) *Survey of the Workload of Public Health Nurses.* Dublin: Institute of Community Health Nursing.

Burnard, P. (1991) A Method of Analysing Interview Transcripts in Qualitative Research, *Nurse Education Today,* 11, 461–6.

Caraher, M. (1994a) A sociological approach to health promotion for nurses in an institutional setting, *Journal of Advanced Nursing,* 20, 544–51.

Caraher, M. (1994b) Nursing and health promotion practice: the creation of victims and winners in a political context, *Journal of Advanced Nursing,* 19, 465–8.

Caraher, M. (1998) Patient education and health promotion: clinical health promotion – the conceptual link, *Patient Education and Counseling,* 33, 49–58.

Catford, J. and Nutbeam, D. (1984) Toward a definition of health education and health promotion, *Health Education Journal,* 43 (2, 3): 38.

Davis, S. (1995) An investigation into nurses' understanding of health education and health promotion within a neuro-rehabilitation setting, *Journal of Advanced Nursing,* 21, 951–9.

Delaney, F. G. (1994) Nursing and health promotion: Conceptual concerns, *Journal of Advanced Nursing,* 20, 828–35.

Department of Health. (1994) *Shaping a Healthier Future: A Strategy for Effective Healthcare in the 1990s.* Dublin: Stationery Office.

Department of Health. (1995) *A Health Promotion Strategy.* Dublin: Department of Health.

Dines, A. and Cribb, A. (1993) *Health Promotion Concepts and Practice.* Oxford: Blackwell.

Donoghue, J., Duffield, C., Pelletier, D., and Adams, A. (1990) Health promotion as a nursing function: perceptions held by university students of nursing, *International Journal of Nursing Studies,* 27 (1): 51–60.

Duncan, D. and Gold, R. S. (1986) Reflections: health promotion – what is it? *Health Values,* 10 (3): 47–8.

Ewles, L. and Simmet, I. (1995) *Promoting Health: A Practical Guide,* 3rd edn. London: Scutari Press.

Glaser, B.G. and Strauss, A.L. (1967) *The Discovery of Grounded Theory. Strategies for Grounded Theory.* New York: Aldine.

Gorin, S.S. (1992) Student nurse opinions about the importance of health promotion practices, *Journal of Community Health,* 17 (6): 367–75.

Gott, M. and O'Brien, M. (1990a) Attitudes and beliefs in health promotion, *Nursing Standard,* 5 (2): 30–2.

Gott, M. and O'Brien, M. (1990b) Practice and the prospect for change, *Nursing Standard,* 5 (3): 30–2.

Gott, M. and O'Brien, M. (1990c) Policy framework for health promotion, *Nursing Standard,* 5 (11): 30–2.

Holcomb, J. D. and Mullen, P. D. (1986) Certified nurse-midwives and health promotion and disease prevention, *Journal of Nurse-Midwifery*, 31 (3): 141–8.

King, P. (1994) Health Promotion: the emerging frontier in nursing, *Journal of Advanced Nursing*, 20, 209–18.

Lask, S., Smith, P., and Masterson, A. (1994) *A curricular review of the pre- and post - registration education programmes for nurses, midwives and health visitors in relation to the integration of a philosophy of health: Developing a model for evaluation*. Research Highlights. London: ENB.

Latter, S. (1993) Health education and health promotion in acute ward settings: nurses perceptions and practice, in: J. Wilson-Barnett and J. MacLeod Clark (eds), *Research in Health Promotion and Nursing*. London: Macmillan.

Latter, S., Macleod Clark, J., Wilson-Barnett, J., and Maben, J. (1992) Health education in nursing: perceptions of practice in acute settings, *Journal of Advanced Nursing*, 17, 164–72.

Lincoln, Y. S. and Guba, E. G. (1985) *Naturalistic Inquiry*. Beverley Hills: Sage.

Maben, J. and Macleod Clark, J. (1995) Health promotion: a concept analysis, *Journal of Advanced Nursing*, 22, 1158–65.

Macleod Clark, J. (1993) From sick nursing to health nursing: evolution or revolution? in: J. Wilson-Barnett and J. Macleod Clark (eds), *Research in Health Promotion and Nursing*. London: Macmillan.

Macleod Clark, J., Haverty, S. and Kendall, S. (1990) Helping people to stop smoking: a study of the nurse's role, *Journal of Advanced Nursing*, 16, 357–63.

Macleod Clark, J. and Maben, J. (1998) Health promotion: perceptions of Project 2000 educated nurses, *Health Education Research*, 13 (2): 185–96.

Macleod Clark, J. and Webb, P. (1985) Health education – a basis for professional practice, *Nurse Education Today*, 5, 210–14

McBride, A. (1994) Health promotion in hospitals: the attitudes, beliefs and practices of hospital nurses, *Journal of Advanced Nursing*, 20, 92–100.

Mahler, H. (1985) Nurses lead the way: health for all through primary health care, *World Health*, July, 28–9.

Melia, K. (1987) *Learning and Working: The Occupational Socialisation of Nurses*. London: Tavistock.

Melvin, B. (1987) Promoting health by example, *Nursing Times*, 83 (17): 42–3.

Mitchinson, S. (1995) A review of the health promotion and health beliefs of traditional and Project 2000 student nurses, *Journal of Advanced Nursing*, 21, 356–63.

Naidoo, J. and Wills, J. (1994) *Health Promotion, Foundation of Practice*. London: Bailliere Tindall.

O'Sullivan, T. (1995) *A Service Without Walls. An Analysis of Public Health Nursing in 1994*. Dublin: Institute of Public Administration.

Parish, R. (1987) Wales paves the way to heart health. *Nursing Times*, 22 April, 34–6.

Patton, M. Q. (1980) *Qualitative Evaluation Methods*. Beverley Hills: Sage.

Piper, S. and Brown, P. (1998) Psychology as a theoretical foundation for health education in nursing: empowerment or social control? *Nurse Education Today*, 18, 637–41.

Robinson, S. and Hill, Y. (1995) Miracles take a little longer: Project 2000 and the health-promoting nurse, *International Journal Nursing Studies*, 32 (6): 568–79.

Sandelowski, M. (1986) The problems of rigor in qualitative research, *Advances in Nursing Science*, 8 (3): 27–37.

Sandelowski, M. (1993) Rigor or rigor mortis: the problem of rigour in qualitative research revisited, *Advances in Nursing Science*, 16 (2): 1–8.

Sandelowski, M. (1998) Focus on qualitative methods. The call to experts in qualitative research, *Research in Nursing and Health*, 21, 467–71.

Sarantakos, S. (1994) *Social Research*. London: Macmillan.

Schultz, P. (1991) Foundations of nursing's perspectives on health education, *Hoitotiede*, 3 (5): 223–30.

Soeken, K., Bausell, R.,Winklestein, M., and Carson, V. J. (1989) Preventive behaviour: attitudes and compliance of nursing students, *Journal of Advanced Nursing*, 14, 1026–33.

Stachtchenko, S. and Jenicek, M. (1990) Conceptual differences between prevention and health promotion: research implications for community health programs, *Canadian Journal of Public Health*, 81, 53–9.

Strauss, A. and Corbin, J. (1990) *Basics of Qualitative Research*. Newbury Park: Sage.

Tones, K. (1993) The theory of health promotion: implications for nursing, in: J. Wilson Barnett and J. Macleod Clark (eds) *Research in Health Promotion and Nursing*. London: Macmillan.

Tones, K., Tilford, S., and Robinson, Y. (1990) *Health Education: Effectiveness and Efficiency*. London: Chapman & Hall.

Treacy, M. (1987) 'In the pipeline': a qualitative study of general nurse training with special reference to nurses' role in health education. Unpublished PhD thesis. University of London.

Treacy, M., Collins, R., Casey, D., and Cooney, A. (1996) Nurses' attitudes related to health promotion activities related to healthy lifestyle – report of a study. Dublin: Department of Nursing Studies, University College Dublin/ Department of Health.

Vincent, M., Fridinger, F., Panhorst, B., and Streater, J. (1985) Health promotion beliefs and practices of a sample of occupational health nurses, *Occupational Health Nursing*, 33, 542–6.

WHO (World Health Organisation) (1986) *Ottawa Charter For Health Promotion: An International Conference on Health Promotion*. Europe: Copenhagen: World Health Organisation Regional Office for Europe.

13

Evaluation Case Study of the Registration/Diploma Nursing Programme

Janice B. Clarke, Mary Gobbi and Helen Simons

INTRODUCTION

This chapter has two aims. The first is to present the methodological justification for implementing a case study approach to the educational evaluation of the 'pilot' Registration/Diploma Programme in Ireland. The second is to illustrate the flexibility of case study design in meeting changing needs in the research field.

The chapter is constructed in three parts. First the scene is set identifying the background to the research problem and the major features of the tender specification. Second, the case study approach is outlined to allow the reader to appreciate its methodological stance and its responsiveness to a changing context. Thirdly, some findings from the study are offered to assist the reader to gain a sense of the outcomes that were generated from the methodological process as described.

SETTING THE SCENE

The case study, which is the focal point of this chapter, was a two-year independent external evaluation of the Registration/Diploma Nursing Programme in Ireland and was commissioned by the Department of Health and Children in collaboration with An Bord Altranais.

During the 1990s, nurse education and training in Ireland experienced a quiet evolution. Its historically rooted, traditional apprenticeship curriculum, which maintained the emphasis of vocation in which the student was predominantly an employee learning on-the-job, was altered to a third level educational model, in which the student became predominantly a supernumerary learner gaining clinical experience in conjunction with receiving an academic education to diploma level.

Despite this major change, it seems that Irish nursing will not stand still for long. The Commission on Nursing (1998) in its Final Report recommended a further move to a four-year degree programme thereby promoting an all graduate profession of nursing in Ireland.

The case study presented in this chapter took place during the historic transition between the traditional Registration and the Registration/ Diploma programme. The evaluation was conducted between May 1996 and May 1998 and focused on the first pilot programme which originated in Galway with its first intake of students in October 1994. When the introduction of the Registration/Diploma programme was announced, Mr Brendan Howlin, the then Minister for Health, indicated that the 'pilot [sites] would be monitored and evaluated before implementation on a national scale' (Howlin, 1994: 5). However, by October 1996, only six months after the evaluation had started, a total of twelve schools of nursing in Ireland had begun the Registration/Diploma based on the Galway model. This left only five general schools of nursing offering the traditional apprenticeship model of training in 1996 and these moved towards the Registration/Diploma programme in October 1997.

The tender specification (Department of Health, 1995) required the evaluation to focus primarily on implementation of the 'new' programme in Galway. The primary aim of the evaluation was to examine the effectiveness in practice of the pilot programme at the Galway site and to ascertain whether the issues identified in Galway were also significant at the sites which began the programme in October 1995. The outcomes would be used to inform future policy making and to provide evidence of how nurses trained under the Registration/Diploma Programme were prepared for the workforce.

The four specific objectives as stated in the tender were:

1 To examine the content, implementation and effects of the programme in practice;
2 To provide interim feedback on the development of the programme;
3 To establish whether the programme meets its objectives, particularly in relation to clinical nursing practice;
4 To consider and document what useful comparisons may be made with the previous apprenticeship model of training (Department of Health, 1995).

This focus on the Galway site remained, despite the changing circumstances owing to the programme's expansion, since Galway was the model on which other programmes were approved. However, in response to the dynamic situation, the evaluation team extended its remit slightly to try to provide evidence beyond the Galway site that would be useful to policy makers for the development of the programme. Towards the end of the two-year evaluation period, issues which had been identified in Galway were discussed with national groups of representatives from 11 other sites, which had started the programme in 1995 and 1996. This process offered evidence as to whether the other sites had experienced similar issues to those identified in Galway thereby offering a firmer foundation for future policy development.

The background to why Ireland should have even considered changing its nurse education and training curriculum is long and complex. Internal and external factors influencing the evolution of the Registration/Diploma Programme in Ireland are well documented in the Final Report of the Independent External Evaluation (Simons et al., 1998). European Union directives were a significant influence on programme design and content (EU Directive 89/595/EEC), the international scene was moving to third-level qualifications in nursing and An Bord Altranais (1991: 13) had agreed that 'Nurse training in its apprenticeship form has had its critics'. An Bord Altranais (1991) had highlighted many reports which led to these conclusions (Bendall, 1973; Fretwell, 1978; Orton, 1980; Reid, 1985) in its own review of nurse education and training which had set out its template in *The Future of Nurse Education and Training in Ireland* (An Bord Altranais, 1994a). Many aspects of An Bord Altranais's report were echoed in the Galway Registration/Diploma programme. A summary of the essential features of the Registration/ Diploma programme is located in Figure 1.

In announcing the introduction of the Registration/Diploma Galway pilot programme in June, 1994, the then Minister for Health, Mr Brendan Howlin, recognised the links that Galway had already established with a third-level institution. In that same speech, the Minister acknowledged the strengths of the traditional programme and indicated his concern that the new programme 'will also have to ensure that the nurse at registration stage will, at the very least, be as competent in a clinical context as her counterpart emerging from the traditional apprenticeship system' (Howlin, 1994).

The concern that a more academically educated nurse might lose some of the qualities already evident in Irish nurses was noted in early interviews in the evaluation. However, both major stakeholders clearly recognised the necessity for change. A spokesperson for An Bord Altranais in February 1997 stated, 'The good nurse idea is not one that will be threatened by the new model. I think that the basic personality trait and the nursing quality, and the understanding of nursing will not change. I believe that what will change is the scope of practice and the things that nurses do.' And a spokesperson from the Department of Health and Children stated in November 1996 that 'you've got to ensure that students are well equipped to deal with the rapidly changing health care scene'.

Figure 1. Essential Features of the Registration/Diploma Programme

- Establishment of a formal link between University College, Galway (UCG) and the School of Nursing to facilitate academic accreditation at Diploma level in conjunction with registration in general or psychiatric nursing with An Bord Altranais.
- Biological and social sciences taught by university teachers from UCG and completed in the first academic year.
- The nursing studies component (two-thirds of the curriculum content) taught by nurse tutors, in block weeks over the two years.
- Throughout their programme, student nurses have university student status and in clinical practice placements, supernumerary status (except for 14 weeks paid rostered service in year three).
- Students nurses have a non means-tested grant from the Western Health Board during the programme (except during rostered service when a salary is received).
- Introduction of Clinical Placement Coordinators to guide and supervise students in their placement areas and to advise, encourage and facilitate students to achieve maximum learning from clinical placements.
- The programme length of 156 weeks which included 4,600 hours of theoretical and clinical instruction in accordance with EU directives 77/452/EEC, 77/453/EEC and 89/595/EEC (Department of Health, 1995).
- The diversity of clinical placements was extended (e.g. to include community and voluntary agencies).
- One week was added to the placement for the care of the elderly.

THE CASE STUDY APPROACH

This section first outlines the background to the case study approach and its application to the remit of the study, clarifies the design generated for this study and highlights the ethical principles and procedures used in the conduct of the evaluation. Secondly the main methods of data gathering are indicated together with the approach taken for analysis and interpretation of evidence. Thirdly, the responsiveness of the case study approach to a changing context is explained with reference to the national issue discussion groups and dearth of stated theoretical and clinical outcomes.

1 Case Study Approach

Case study is the study of a single instance, institution or programme. It is adopted when it is important to understand complex social phenomena within particular contexts, retaining the 'holistic and meaningful character-istics of real-life events' in the context in which they occur (Yin, 1989: 14).

One of the basic arguments for a case study approach in evaluation (Simons, 1980; Stake, 1995) is that it allows for the complexity and impact of the programmes to be documented in context through the experiences of participants, in relation to issues identified by them and by key stakeholders. Robson (1993: 52) encapsulates this in his definition of case study: 'Case study is a strategy for doing research which involves an empirical investigation of a particular contemporary phenomenon within its real life context using multiple sources of evidence'. The important points Robson highlights are that case study is more of a strategy than a method; it is empirical in that it relies on the collection of evidence about what is going on; it is about the particular, the specific case which demands caution in generalisation; it focuses on the phenomenon in context where there may be a merger between the two; and it requires the use of multiple methods and sources for the collection of evidence.

1.1 Application and design
Justification that the case study approach or strategy was particularly appropriate for evaluating the Registration/Diploma Programme in Galway is outlined in Figure 2 (Simons et al., 1998). The aim of the case study of the Galway site was to capture the reality of implementation of the Registration/Diploma Programme in context to provide a database to inform future development and policy making. The evaluation design that emerged set the process for this aim to be realised. The primary focus of the case study was on the general programme (consideration was given to the psychiatric Registration/Diploma programme which was introduced with a cohort of 12 students in October 1995 but did not constitute an evaluation in itself). The main design feature of the Galway case study was supported initially by five other design components:

- in-depth profiles of the experience of a sample of students and clinical placements coordinators in the Registration/Diploma Programme
- a series of interviews with the major stakeholders in nurse education and training in Ireland
- analysis of research and literature relevant to nurse education and training in Ireland
- observation of classroom teaching and students in practice placements to reveal the programme in action and outcome
- analysis of a sample of student nurses taking part in the programme compared to those trained on the previous apprenticeship model

In the event it was not possible to undertake the last component listed as the apprenticeship model was gradually eroded with further schools of

Figure 2. Justification for Use of Case Study for the Independent External Evaluation of the Registration/Diploma Progamme in Galway

---

- The programme was a pilot study at its inception, the first of its kind in Ireland. It was accepted by the Department of Health as model for other institutions to follow. Given this fact and intention, it was essential to provide detailed documentation of its process and outcomes to inform future development of the Registration/Diploma Programme.

- The Registration/Diploma Programme was a major departure from the traditional model of education and training and its effects were unknown. It was important to study these in depth and over time. The case study approach allows for this flexibility.

- Several institutions and stakeholders had an interest in this major change in nurse education and training. The case study approach allowed the evaluation to portray multiple perspectives, respond to different concerns of stakeholders and document the complexity of the programme in practice

- The case study approach is sensitive to contexts. By presenting data interpreted in context, future developers of the programme would be able to decide which issues were specific to the site of Galway and which had resonance for them in their own context

---

nursing adopting the Registration/Diploma Programme. The traditional student groups in Galway had ceased to exist by the time the evaluation started, as Galway had already adapted its curriculum model in 1992.

Two additional design features were later added: the first to extend the database in the case study, the second to strengthen the claims for the findings generated from the case.

- short questionnaire to a sample of outgoing students (the first cohort) from the Galway site, ward sisters and clinical placement coordinators to gauge student learning outcomes
- issue discussion groups towards the end of the second year to ascertain whether the issues identified in the Galway case study were also significant in other sites across Ireland

These two additions will be considered in the third section (see p. 216), concerning the responsive nature of the case study approach but, first, the ethical procedures concerning the conduct of the evaluation will be addressed.

1.2 Ethical procedures

Ethical procedures are important in any research with the overriding imperative 'to do no harm'. A major guiding principle is 'a respect for confidentiality and the anonymity of informants and advisers' (Daniel, 1993: 14). In case study evaluation, where it is often not possible to anonymise participants and where individuals may have different perceptions of what took place and different interests in the outcomes, an ethical code of conduct is essential for the gathering and sharing of information.

Ethical principles and procedures for the conduct of the evaluation were thoroughly discussed for consensus within the evaluation team. Guidelines produced by Simons (1988) provided the basis for the procedures and these were further developed using the International Council of Nursing Guidelines (1996). These guidelines were based on the principles of confidentiality, impartiality, negotiation and independence for the conduct of the fieldwork and processing and clearance in reporting. The agreed ethical procedures were made available to all personnel involved in the evaluation and discussed with them prior to interview or observation to clarify the conduct of the fieldwork, mutual commitments to the evaluation and plans for distribution of reports. Three criteria of reporting which encapsulated the ethical principles were accuracy, relevance of the content to the research goals and fairness.

Access to personnel can be a sensitive issue in case study evaluation and so the principle of double access was employed. Permission was initially sought from the gatekeepers (major stakeholders) and secondly from individuals themselves before evidence was sought. Gaining access through formal channels is not an immediate recommendation that all individuals should agree to be interviewed or observed without further clarification of their involvement, how the data will be used and how the findings will be reported. Further negotiation may be required and additional procedures generated if the need arises.

2 Collection of Evidence

Eight major methods were employed in the case study for the collection of evidence. These are presented in Figure 3. Interviews and observation require some further explanation as they (together with analysis of documents) were the dominant methods employed.

Interviews

Interview schedules were developed and were based on issues identified in preliminary stakeholder interviews and available literature on nurse education and training in Ireland. These schedules were constantly refined and refocused as the evaluation progressed. Both individual and

Figure 3 Methods Employed for Data Collection

- individual in-depth interviews
- group in-depth interviews
- case profiles of individual students and clinical placement coordinators
- recorded observations, both clinical and classroom
- analysis of documentation (published and unpublished)
- short questionnaire
- self-evaluation in the case study site
- fieldwork notes from site visits

group interviews in the initial stages of the evaluation were open-ended to gain participants' perspectives on issues they considered important for the evaluation to pursue. As these were confirmed as significant, the interview questions became more semi-structured and later structured to pursue in-depth understanding. All interviews were tape-recorded where permission was given and the majority were transcribed. This process was to promote accuracy of reporting, to support analysis and interpretation and to lend veracity to the reporting.

Observations
Observations were of three kinds: general observations on site to inform the evaluation team's understanding of the Galway context; classroom observations where feasible; and clinical observations first, when the students were supernumerary, secondly, towards the end of their third year when on rostered service, and thirdly, when the recently registered nurses from the first cohort were observed on the wards as staff nurses. Observational data did not form a major part of the case study due to some difficulties beyond the control of the evaluation (see Simons et al., 1998) and so were mainly used to cross-reference and support data gained from interviews and analysis of documents.

2.1. Analysis and interpretation of evidence
Robson (1993: 162) suggests that the quality of a case study depends 'to a great extent on the quality of the investigator' and that case study research requires well trained and experienced investigators. He also identifies five other skills: an enquiring mind for question asking, good listening ability, adaptiveness and flexibility to respond to the unexpected, grasp of the issues during the course of the study and lack of bias to allow openness to contrary findings. In this evaluation the team approach was an added advantage. It increased the reliability of the findings as perceptions

were frequently cross-validated; members of the team were involved in all stages from beginning to end through frequent discussion, refocusing of interviews, negotiation and also in checking and re-checking of draft reports for eventual agreement.

Analysis was a continuing process which involved all members of the team from the inception of the study, to the choice of interview questions and issues to pursue, methods to adopt, individuals to interview and the progressive focusing of issues. Yet it was also possible to identify a systematic process that was utilised to make sense of all the evidence collected. This involved examining all the interview transcripts, field notes and observations for key analytical themes, categorising these, triangulating with other evidence from other sources, searching for patterns in the themes, and interpreting and presenting evidence to illuminate the key questions and aims of the study. Six stages were identified in this process (Simons et al., 1998) as presented in Figure 4.

Figure 4. Six Stage Analysis Process

---

1 The interview data, field notes and relevant documentation were read by all members of the team and issues identified as significant to an understanding of the programme.

2 These were triangulated, that is, each was analysed to see if it was supported by data from other sources and other people.

3 The significance of the issues was then re-examined in the light of evidence arising from further site visits and issues were reformulated as necessary to reflect a greater understanding of the case.

4 Stage four involved exploring the interrelationship between the issues to see what patterns were beginning to emerge.

5 Stage five involved searching the whole database once again for evidence to support the emerging findings.

6 Finally the issues and findings which were identified consistently and had sufficient data to verify their significance for an understanding of the programme in practice were included in the report and implications highlighted in the final chapter.

In order to report the evidence reasonably and fairly, no issue was recognised as significant unless reported by at least three participants (in most cases it was more than three). In reporting the issue as a finding, sometimes only one quotation was offered to support the point, although more were in the data base. Usually the quotation is only one of a number that could have been selected.

3 Responsiveness of the Case Study Approach

When the situation under study changes during an investigation, or information that one would anticipate finding is not present, it is useful to be able to adapt the research approach to accommodate such changes and gain evidence to support future policy decisions. Two main areas evoked such a response in this case study. The first was the unexpected absence of any documented curriculum outlining the programme's philosophy, aims, content or outcomes. (However, a Galway course document was made available in the summer of 1997, nine months before the evaluation ended.) The second was that the Galway site did not remain the only pilot site for long. As already stated, by 1996 only five general schools of nursing still offered the traditional apprenticeship model of training and these moved towards the Registration/Diploma programme by October 1997. Both of these situations were responded to by the evaluation team.

It may be recalled that the last two specific objectives in the tender document for the evaluation involved establishing whether the programme met its objectives, particularly in relation 'to clinical practice and to consider and document what useful comparisons may be made with the previous apprenticeship model of training' (Department of Health, 1995). In the initial absence of any curriculum outcomes and the continued absence of any specific theoretical or clinical learning outcomes, it was not possible to track student development explicitly from the outset in relation to locally derived criteria, Alternative indicators had to be sought. First, criteria and competencies derived from An Bord Altranais (1994a) and competencies identified by the WHO (1991) provided the background criteria for gathering data. Second, to appreciate the Irish context, the evaluation team documented interview evidence from a range of participants in relation to perceived qualities of the 'good Irish nurse' trained through the apprenticeship system together with desired attributes of nurses for the future. Information from these strategies enabled the evaluation team to frame their investigation and explore the ongoing progress of the students with these in mind.

Four indicators of student performance were also utilised towards the end of the evaluation. The first was evidence of the students' theoretical achievements and clinical nursing skills from the examination systems of An Bord Altranais and University College Galway (renamed National University of Ireland, Galway, 16 June 1997). The second was evidence related to the course objectives (which were made available in the summer of 1997) through observation of practice and a short questionnaire to outgoing students, ward sisters and clinical placement coordinators. The third was from interview evidence with ward sisters, staff nurses, nurse managers and nurse tutors who commented on the students' performance during rostered service and when they began practising as registered nurses. The fourth was direct observation of six members of the first cohort who were practising as part-time staff nurses while on the full-time fourth year of the degree programme.

The second change – the extension of the 'pilot' to all sites in Ireland – led to two major changes to the research design. First the comparison of a sample of Registration/Diploma students with traditional students had to be dropped. Second was the introduction of national issue-discussion groups (an extension of the original remit) to explore the extent to which the issues identified in the Galway site were also significant in sites that introduced the Registration/Diploma Programme in 1995 and 1996. The discussion groups were held in Dublin in March 1998 with representatives from all sites then participating in the programme, other than Galway and three other sites which had previously been visited. One of the disadvantages often cited of the case study approach is the potential difficulty of generalising from the single case, and, in the policy context, of knowing to what extent the issues in the case may be idiosyncratic to that site. The introduction of issue discussion groups at the national level enabled the evaluation to test the degree to which the issues identifiable in the case site were represented in a larger population. The order in which these took place is important. The case study was undertaken first. Hence the issues were well grounded in the context of the case. This use of case study data in extension for other sites supports concerns about the generalisability of single case study outcomes and the usefulness of the findings for policy (Robson, 1993).

At this stage in the chapter, it seems appropriate to close the research circle and offer the reader illustrations of some research outcomes gained through the case study evaluation.

FOUR FINDINGS

Introduction

Seven major categories of findings were presented in the Final Report of the evaluation to the commissioning agents in conjunction with associated implications (Simons et al., 1998) The categories were as follows: curriculum (including pedagogy), assessment, students' experience (including supernumerary status, clinical coordinators' experience and financial hardship), partnership, staff preparation and development and finally the psychiatric experience. A finding from each of the first three categories will be briefly considered to give a sense of how findings were constructed from the evidence.

The first two findings on curriculum and assessment illustrate the context in which the curriculum was designed: the political, ideological, professional and pragmatic influences which shaped its structure, and the factors which impinged upon its delivery and the way the students experienced the programme. During the period of the evaluation, the Registration/Diploma Programme was required to operate within the context of existing An Bord Altranais Rules which influenced curriculum content, the assessment of clinical nursing skills and specified details concerning the assessment of theoretical knowledge.[1] In particular, An Bord Altranais assessment requirements during the first 52 weeks of the programme had a marked effect. The third-level institute, in this case the National University of Ireland, Galway, operated within a tradition in which each theoretical subject was assessed, usually by examination, by the Faculty delivering the tuition. In order to ascertain the rationale behind the planned and implemented curriculum and assessment processes it was necessary to interview those who had been involved in the initial design phases at both a strategic policy and implementation level. Scrutiny of meeting notes and internal reports revealed the difference between *intent* and the *reality* of the implemented curriculum. Often it was difficult to triangulate perceptions and memories of the decision-making processes, especially where these differed and where the written record itself was contested. In these circumstances, differing perspectives were respected and recorded.

Finding 1: *There were differences of opinion concerning the nature, purpose and scheduling of tuition in the biological and social sciences.*
Capturing the 'live' or 'experienced' curriculum in the absence of sub-stantive documentation required a cyclical pattern of investigation, triangulation and verification whether through interview, observation or documentary analysis. Where respondents offered differing reports, perceptions and judgements concerning key events, the researchers had a particular responsibility to adhere to the ethical principles and pro-cedures of fairness, accuracy and relevance in reporting and report these differences. *Differences* between respondents can be as significant as *similarities* as Finding 1 states.

These differences identified ideological and pragmatic stances concerning the nature of nursing as a practice-based discipline and the contribution of other disciplinary subjects to its learning and development. The 'Galway' model was predicated upon a particular relationship between the first year and the remainder of the programme. During this first year, approximately 36 per cent of the curriculum hours are assigned to the biological and social sciences, although as a proportion of the *total curriculum* hours they comprise only 10.6 per cent. One effect of this distribution of hours was that students experienced a first year dominated by theoretical tuition and numerous assessments in the biological and social sciences. According to the course document and the University Calendar, the first year was conceived as:

> [A] Foundation Year which will equip the nursing student with the desirable levels of knowledge in relevant sciences. It places strong emphasis on giving a sound biological and social science base. In addition, the range of courses involved, which are closely related to those taken by students of other disciplines, will ensure adequate integration of the nursing students with the general body of university students from the beginning. (UCG Calendar, 1995/6: 439, para. 2.3).

In effect, for philosophical, pragmatic and financial reasons, the tuition of the biological and social sciences was restricted to the first year of the Programme. University teachers questioned the appropriateness of their subjects being restricted to the first year, as one argued: 'It's not easy to deliver pharmacology very early in the course. It's dependent upon physiology and pathophysiology in order to have relevance to what the students are going to do'. The relevance of the tuition, its sequence in relation to the students' clinical practice and tuition in other subjects like applied genetics, embryology, and applied sociology were raised by other respondents. Several university teachers indicated that it was not additional time that they required, rather 'the opportunity to come back later once the students have had some practical experience'.

Whether the biological and social sciences were to be delivered and assessed as 'foundation', 'introductory,' 'applied' or 'pure' subjects similar to those of other university students was another source of tension. These various perspectives influenced judgements concerning who should be the most appropriate person to teach and assess the individual subjects. Several university teachers and nurse tutors echoed the views of this quotation from a university teacher who questioned: 'What was wrong with the nurse tutors who were doing the anatomy and physiology teaching originally?'

Some university teachers tried to make their subjects 'real' for the students, but considered that 'it's not real as far as nursing goes', a view acknowledged by those nurse tutors who reported that students 'have straight lectures from the "ologist" who does not apply it to nursing', and therefore they had to 'revisit' subjects later in the programme. A similar perspective was articulated by students, for example 'the lectures were sometimes not relevant to nursing'. In contrast, there were nurse tutors and ward sisters who noted that students 'see the relevance' and 'importance' of the pure sciences in their second and third years, an observation which is supported by student comments in the student experience category.

Examination of course materials, calendar entries and interviews with university teachers, nurse tutors and students indicate that there were perceived differences of interpretation and uncertainties as to the purpose of biological and social sciences tuition and disagreement as to who should have control over the curriculum. Strategically, other issues emerged, for example the extent to which there could be shared teaching with other university students, whether students' work should be marked or moderated by nurse tutors, whether the teachers of the biological and social sciences should have expertise/experience in health care settings, and whether the tuition should be integrated within clinically focused topics or continue to be delivered as discrete subjects. These contrasting reports illustrate the political and ideological nature of curriculum design and assessment and demonstrate the usefulness of case study and evaluative methodologies which enable a multi-layered and sometimes complex picture to be portrayed.

Finding 2: *An Bord Altranais Rules and practices governing the management of practice-based assessments required for registration purposes were considered inappropriate for Registration/Diploma students in relation to professional practice. Many course objectives and desired competencies of the students were not amenable to assessment through the Proficiency Assessment Form (PAF)*

The second finding demonstrated that not only did existing difficulties experienced with An Bord Altranais's method of assessment of clinical nursing skills continue with the Registration/Diploma, but that new problems emerged.

The Proficiency Assessment Form was designed for the apprenticeship training and applied in each clinical setting in which the student was assessed and for all branches of the register. The form comprises eight dimensions of practice with their sub-division criteria. Each criterion is rated on a four point scale, with one being the best mark possible. When the course document objectives of the Registration/Diploma Programme were compared with the PAF criteria it became apparent that the PAF did not assess the range of attributes expected in the Registration/ Diploma Programme. Furthermore, the PAF had not been designed to cater for the new clinical settings in which students were gaining experience (e.g. hospice, community). One nurse tutor remarked in 1996, 'An Bord Altranais regulations were set in a different era. I don't even think they match that era. They don't fit in at all with what's happening now.'

Existing criticisms of the PAF system were echoed by students, ward sisters, staff nurses, senior nurse managers and nurse tutors, namely that there were problems with marking, discrimination, consistency and a tendency not to give students poor marks (see McSweeney, 1995 for a more detailed analysis of the PAF). These examples from ward sisters are typical of the comments received: 'However much you try you could not give them a 3 or 4 [low marks]; 'there are some born nurses who cannot shine on these forms'; and 'the mediocre ones really, they are not bad enough for a three or a four, there have been a few that you are not totally happy with, but you know if you read the comments they are not a 3 or 4'. In addition some ward sisters considered that the clinical assessment scheme should have been changed for the Registration/ Diploma and adjusted for students at different stages in the programme. A typical comment from a ward sister was that it was 'ridiculous' to assess a student at the end of her first six weeks in practice in relation to her capacity to 'direct and work with a junior'. The necessity to use the PAF system meant that if a school of nursing were to assess the range of attributes and competencies expected of the Registration/Diploma student, then they would need to devise an additional assessment tool to that of the PAF. During the national issue discussion groups it became apparent that some Schools of Nursing had devised additional assessment strategies to the PAF. There were several implications from this finding including a reappraisal of An Bord Rules, which is currently in progress. It was suggested that a review of the PAF was urgently needed and that such a review should examine (among other things) whether a national assessment tool could be designed to be appropriate for each clinical setting and any curriculum model; whether third-level institutions should be involved in the assessment of clinical skills; and whether it is appropriate to establish national standards or competencies for registration purposes which could be incorporated into a range of assessment models. These implications present an opportunity for policy makers to extend their debate on the future of nurse education and training in Ireland.

Finding 3: *Students reported that practice was the main catalyst for their learning*
In the first 36 weeks of the Programme which were theoretical, students complained that they perceived much of the theoretical instruction not to be relevant to nursing which made it more difficult to learn and assimilate the knowledge. Once in practice, however, they were able to make sense of clinical situations and utilise knowledge more effectively drawing on previous theoretical instruction to assist practice and using practice to understand subsequent theory. Three groups of students were tracked during the course of the case study evaluation. Written reflective profiles and interviews were conducted on every site visit with three groups of students (n=14) from the October 1994 and 1995 cohorts to offer a time trajectory of their experiences.

A student just completing her first year of the programme wrote in November 1996: 'I think I have learned more from incidents that happen in the clinical area than from what we are taught in class. Actually working on the ward and dealing with a specific patient and his/her problem or illness tends to stick in your mind more. I also think we get plenty of opportunities while we are on the ward'. However, a second-year student was able to reflect back on the subjects taught in the first year and remark how she and her colleagues were recognising the value of the subjects they had been studying, 'You don't think at the time that they're any good but when you get on the ward you think, "Oh yes, I know, we were doing this"' to which another student adds, 'You're just thinking you'll never ever use this and then, I think it's very good now. I'm glad we've had the chance to do those subjects.'

The importance of learning in the clinical areas was clearly stated by a qualified Registration/Diploma nurse in March 1998 when she summarised her own perspective (which was supported by colleagues) that theory, 'means nothing when you haven't been on a ward'. The implications of this finding are that given the strength of learning through practice, it would be helpful if earlier clinical experience could be time-tabled and the relevance of practice emphasised more in theoretical tuition.

Finding 4 *The clinical placement coordinators (CPCs) made an enormous contribution to student learning*
The CPC role was introduced for the Registration/Diploma Programme to allocate and support supernumerary students in clinical areas. This innovation was overwhelmingly supported in the Galway case study site. Students found it particularly helpful when, 'they do total patient care with us, go right through a patient and then in the afternoon they might come back and they take us all together and they might go through something with us'. (First-year student, July 1996)

In November 1996, a profile student clarified: 'They have encouraged us to use our initiative and research certain topics which are of value to us'. Eight months later, in July 1997, she wrote, 'The clinical coordinators are most influential to me in this programme. They have taught and encouraged us to be assertive, question certain practices and to stand up for both our rights and those of our patients.' Even as third-year students, the support and influence of the CPC's was felt by students: 'We say to the coordinators that we don't know anything and they say you know loads, sometimes you need someone else to see what you know . . . They worked with us from the beginning so they notice things' (March 1997).

However, in the national issue discussion groups, which did not include student representatives, there was an alternative view that the role of CPC's was ambiguous and perhaps temporary while the Programme was new. A nurse tutor when referring to CPCs said: 'I find great difficulty with them – not personally but with their role'. A Director of Nursing added, 'the CPC role will become more evident as the programme progresses'. Since nationally there were differences in the perception of utility of CPC roles and different ways in which the role was practised, it was suggested that 'their role should be [further] discussed in order to build on what works'.

The main implication related to this finding was that if the CPC role is the preferred model for supporting learning in the clinical environment, then the temporary nature of the role should be reviewed in the light of several points which are made in the Independent External Evaluation Final Report. These include greater clarity of the role, a question whether there was a need for national prescription or local flexibility for the role specification, clarity regarding ratios between CPCs and students and a possible career structure for CPCs. If the role was not to be retained, then continuing professional development for staff nurses needed to be reviewed.

CONCLUSION

The 'doing of research' in the real world may offer the researchers situations which are unpredictable and unsolicited. In light of this probability, case study design offers researchers the flexibility to accommodate unplanned obstacles or changing circumstances but still remain close to the initial questions and produce findings to support policy makers. This chapter has presented evidence in support of its two aims: first, justification of the methodological stance of a case study approach for the educational evaluation of the Registration/Diploma curriculum in Ireland and second in illustrating how case study design offers flexibility. In support of these aims, aspects from four findings have been presented to make the connection between the case study evaluation process and its outcomes.

NOTE

1 See The Nurses Act (1985), *Nurses Rules* (An Bord Altranais, 1988 and subsequent amendments), An Bord Altranais Syllabus (1993) and An Bord Altranais *Rules for the Education and Training of Student Nurses* (1994b).

REFERENCES

Bendall, E. (1973) The relationship between recall and application of learning in trainee nurses, PhD thesis, University of London.

An Bord Altranais (1988) *Nurses Rules 1988 and Subsequent Amendments* made under the Nurses Act 1985. Dublin: Stationery Office.

An Bord Altranais (1991) *Nurse Education and Training Consultative Document: Interim*

Report of the Review Committee on Nurse Education and Training. Dublin: An
    Bord Altranais.
An Bord Altranais (1993) *Syllabus for the Education and Training of Student Nurses
    General*, 2nd edn. Dublin: Stationery Office.
An Bord Altranais (1994a) *The Future of Nurse Education and Training in Ireland*.
    Dublin: An Bord Altranais.
An Bord Altranais (1994b) *Rules for the Education and Training of Student Nurses*.
    Dublin: An Bord Altranais.
Commission on Nursing (1998) *Final Report: A Blueprint for the Future*. Dublin:
    Stationery Office.
Daniel, A. (1993) Sampling: purpose and generality, in: D. Colquhoun and A.
    Kellehear (eds), *Health Research in Practice: Political, Ethical and Methodological
    Issues*. London: Chapman & Hall.
Department of Health (1995) *Background to Proposal for Evaluation of Registration/
    Diploma Programme*, August 1995, Briefing Document, Memo.
Fretwell, J. (1978) Socialisation of nurse teaching and learning in hospital wards.
    Unpublished PhD thesis. University of Warwick.
Howlin, B. (1994) *Address by Mr Brendan Howlin TD, Minister for Health on the
    occasion of the presentation of the Bord Altranais report on the future of Nurse Education
    and Training in Ireland*. Notes from Ministerial Address, 29 June 1994.
International Council of Nurses (1996) *Better Health Through Nursing Research*.
    Geneva: ICN
McSweeney (1995) Measurement of nursing skills. Unpublished MEd Dissertation.
    University of Wales: Bangor.
Nurses Act (1985) (No. 18 of 1985), Dublin: Stationery Office.
Orton, H.D. (1980) Ward learning climate and student nurse response. Unpublished
    MPhil thesis. Sheffield Polytechnic.
Reid N (1985) *Wards in Chancery Lane*. London: Royal College of Nursing.
Robson, C. (1993) *Real World Research*. Oxford: Blackwell.
Simons, H. (ed.) (1980) *Towards a Science of the Singular: essays about Case Study in
    Educational Research and Evaluation*. Occasional Publications No 10. Norwich:
    University of East Anglia.
Simons, H. (1988) Ethics of case study in educational research and evaluation, in: R.
    Burgess (ed.), *The Ethics of Educational Research*. Lewes: Falmer Press.
Stake, R.E. (1995) *The Art of Case Study Research*. London: Sage.
University College Galway (1997) *Calendars 1995/6*.
Simons, H., Clarke, J.B., Gobbi, M., and Long, G. (1998) *Nurse Education and
    Training Evaluation in Ireland: Independent External Evaluation*. Dublin: Stationery
    Office.
WHO (World Health Organisation) (1991) *Reviewing and Reorienting the Basic
    Nursing Curriculum*. (Health for All Nursing Series, No. 4), Copenhagen:
    WHO Regional Office for Europe.
Yin, R.K, (1989) *Case Study Research*. London: Sage.

14

Student Midwives' Experiences During Their Training Programme

Cecily M. Begley

INTRODUCTION

Over the past century there has been an increase in hospitalisation for normal births throughout the Western world (Wagner, 1994) and in Ireland home births have decreased from 20 per cent in 1961 (Department of Health, 1976) to five per cent in 1996 (Wiley and Merriman, 1996). This increase in the medicalisation of childbirth has been described as leading to a diminution of the midwife's role (Donnison, 1988; Murphy-Lawless 1998). Studies of midwives' provision of care in Ireland have not shown them to be fulfilling their role in the fullest sense (Byrne, 1989; Coleman, 1989). In particular, midwives in some hospitals act more as obstetric nurses than as autonomous practitioners.

LITERATURE REVIEW

Although there had been a number of studies investigating the world of the student nurse (Melia, 1981; Treacy, 1987; Seed, 1991), very little work had been carried out examining the lives of student midwives. One small qualitative study of student midwives in the United Kingdom in their first three months of training showed that although they were given the rhetoric about midwives being 'practitioners in their own right' in the classroom, the reality they experienced on the wards was very different (Davies, 1990). A larger quantitative study in the UK looked specifically at the adequacy of students' education prior to the introduction of the new 18-month programme (Golden, 1980). This work was continued by Robinson (1986) who looked at student midwives' views of their education.

No major studies had been carried out previously into midwifery education in Ireland but a small study of Irish midwives examined their role in clinical decision making. This showed that while some midwives do contest decisions made by obstetricians, such direct confrontation is not often sought and one of the midwives' main roles was to act as intermediary, or 'piggy in the middle' between the woman and the obstetrician (Murphy-Lawless, 1991). These results have obvious implications for the education of student midwives.

The research presented in this chapter addressed the need for a study into Irish midwifery education by examining the perceptions of student midwives of their working and learning world.

AIM OF STUDY

The study was designed to explore the opinions, feelings and views of student midwives as they progressed through their two-year training in Ireland. The main aim was to interpret and understand the working and learning world of the participants with a view to assisting future students to improve their educational experiences.

METHODS

The methods, instruments and conduct of this study have been described in detail in previous publications (Begley, 1997; Begley, 1999a), so only a brief synopsis is presented here. In the full study (Begley, 1996), the technique of triangulation was employed in a number of ways in an attempt to ensure confirmation and completeness of data. Both quantitative and qualitative methods were used, the quantitative section of the study taking a survey approach, using two questionnaires which were administered to the total population in their first week in the programme and two to three months prior to completion, respectively. The qualitative section of the study involved diary-keeping, interviews and focus group interviews. A pilot study was carried out and changes made as necessary.

Population

Ethical approval and permission for the study to be carried out was granted by the Matrons and Principal Tutors of all seven of the midwifery schools in Southern Ireland. The population, of 125 participants, consisted of all students in the first intake of 1995 in every midwifery school in Ireland. All participants were female. The students were informed of the purpose and proposed conduct of the study and all agreed to participate. Fifty of the students were included in the main qualitative section, 19 of them choosing to keep an unstructured diary and 31 of them volunteering to be interviewed. All students were involved in the focus group interviews.

Instruments

Nineteen volunteers kept unstructured diaries for the first three to ten weeks of their clinical experience. Thirty-one students took part in unstructured interviews three times during the course of their educational programme at four, 12 and 20 months. Focus group interviews were conducted, with the students' permission, following the completion of the final questionnaire when the students were 21–22 months into their programme.

The initial questionnaire sought information on demographic details, preconceptions and future plans. The questions forming the main part of the final questionnaire were derived from the qualitative data, utilising sequential triangulation (Field and Morse, 1985), and the findings served to confirm the qualitative data. Information was gathered also on the students' views of the amount and quality of the theoretical course content. All questionnaires were pre-tested on a group of five midwives prior to the pilot study which involved eleven student midwives.

Data Collection

Interviews took place mainly in the students' homes. The individual interviews lasted from 15 to 76 minutes with a mean of 35 minutes (S.D. 11); group interviews lasted between 30 and 70 minutes. All interviews were tape-recorded and, when transcribed, resulted in a total of 451,649 words.

The 19 diaries returned had been kept from three to ten weeks. They generated between them a total of 19,151 words, with the shortest diary having 254 words and the longest having 2,638 words, a mean of 1,008 (S.D. 768) words. All data were kept strictly confidential by using pseudonyms for the participants and identifying letters for the hospitals.

Qualitative Data Analysis

The interviews and diaries were transcribed, copied into the software programme 'Ethnograph'[1] and subjected to initial analysis, during which 163 codes were assigned. A phenomenological approach was applied to guide data analysis, using the 'description and interpretation' approach of the Dutch school (Holloway and Wheeler, 1996) and eight themes emerged from the data within the diaries and first interviews. A further four themes were identified from the data gleaned from the second interviews.

The 'thick description' of these 12 themes was sent to all 50 students who had taken part in the qualitative section of the study and they were asked to read the interpretation of the selected quotes and to answer a verification questionnaire. Thirty-one (62 per cent) and 29 (58 per cent) students responded in relation to the preliminary results of the first interview and diary data and the second interview data, respectively. The results showed that between 23 (79 per cent) and 31 (100 per cent) of those who replied agreed that a particular theme was either 'very' or 'fairly' true to life. Three further themes were identified from the data arising from the third and group interviews and verification of these themes was undertaken during the final questionnaire only as the students were approaching their final examinations.

The findings have been discussed in full in an unpublished document (Begley, 1997), and under certain specific headings in a number of published papers (Begley, 1998; 1999b; 1999c). A brief synopsis will be presented here under four headings describing respondents' demographic details and the students' views on their education, working role and relationships with staff.

QUALITATIVE FINDINGS AND DISCUSSION

1 Demographic Details

One hundred and twenty-two students (97.6 per cent) completed the first questionnaire (three were ill on the day of distribution). All were registered nurses aged from 21 to 39 years with a mean age of 24 years, seven months (S.D. 2.64). They had six months to 17 years' clinical experience, with an average of two years, seven months in practice (S.D.= 2.18). Four of the students were married. Five had one child each, aged one year (two students), two years (two students) and three years (one student).

The ages of those who offered to keep diaries (25 years, four months (S.D.= 3.83)) or to be interviewed (24 years, three months (S.D.= 1.83)) did not differ significantly from those who did neither (24 years, six months (S.D.= 2.53)), using the Kruskal–Wallis analysis of variance test (F=1.238, p=0.54, d.f.=121).

One hundred and nineteen respondents completed the final questionnaire; six had left midwifery training.

2 Student Midwives' Views of Their Education

'We're workers, not learners'
The majority of students, from all hospitals, commented that they were seen to be there in order to work and that their role as students was seldom, if ever, recognised:

+Jo, 6 July 1995, 1st int., A, 46–52
You go onto the wards at eight o'clock and you do not stop running until
half four, and you're still not looking after anybody properly. And there's
no interest in teaching you or anything else . . . it's a real shock to the
system.

Student midwives in Ireland are all full-time employees, but there did
seem to be little or no acknowledgement of their learner status. This
'worker' status has been documented in other studies of Irish (Treacy,
1987; Coughlan, 1995) and United Kingdom (Melia, 1981; Seed, 1991;
May et al, 1997) general nurse and midwifery education.

A lack of clinical teaching has also been identified in other studies also
(Treacy, 1987; Robinson, 1991; Wilson and Startup, 1991; Raymond
and Ananda-Rajan, 1993; Chamberlain, 1997) and contributes to the
theory/practice divide which has been well documented in the nursing
and midwifery literature (Alexander, 1983; McCaugherty, 1991; Ashworth
and Longmate; 1993). Greenwood (1993) believes that this divide will
continue for as long as nurse (or midwife) teachers remain chiefly in the
classroom. He recommends that they should work alongside students in
the clinical area, a view supported by McCaugherty (1991) who
advocates clinical patient-based tutorials as an excellent way to bridge
the theory-practice gap. Chamberlain (1997) also states that midwife
teachers need to rediscover what it is like to be a clinical midwife in
order to teach a more realistic approach to care.

Overcrowding and working with less than the optimum staff were
also problems identified, which led to extreme tiredness in the students:

+Valerie, diary, D, 72–75
I am totally and utterly limp and exhausted. I thought 13 hr days were
illegal. I can't walk any more, and my shoulders are so tensed that they're
up round my ears . . .

Wards where the physical workload is excessive have been identified as
poor quality learning environments (Smith, 1987). In the present study,
even when the wards were quiet the students could not study or talk
with the women in their care; often they were sent on 'relief' to other
wards, sometimes to areas where they had no previous experience.

'Getting the hang of it'
By the time the students had completed their first four months of
midwifery education they expressed the view that they were 'getting the
hang of' midwifery. With increasing knowledge and confidence came a
sense of achievement:

+Alice, 2 Aug 1995, 1st int., E, 569–577, 579–587
. . . but I really got in with her, I was getting the back going, I was
getting her up onto the commode, I got the pethedine, I had her

breathing properly, she was using the gas well and she was making it and I thought God, like I couldn't do this four months ago . . . I was telling her what to do, I was there with her, I was rubbing the back and, like, she got such immense relief from it, I thought you know this is incredible – people say 'rub your back' and I'm thinking 'where, how, when?'. And here I'm doing it and she's getting great relief from it.

'It's a do-it-yourself course'

Midwifery students in Southern Ireland have at this time (June 1999) only 13 weeks of theoretical input so that a large portion of the course has, perforce, to be studied in the students' free time. The students described this as 'do-it-yourself' learning, without much support from the teaching staff. In some of the schools the students were left for long periods with no set work to do, nor the freedom to leave the classroom to study in the library:

+Amy, 19 March 1996, 2nd int., B, 623–631
Well, a lot of the time you spend in block to be honest with you is a waste of time. We go in every morning and we start at half past eight and our first lecture is at half past ten. We do nothing from half past eight 'til ten o'clock, we sit there every single morning, we do – nothing (eyebrows raised, nodding).

When students have no control over the time they spend in studying it demonstrates the power that teachers have over them (Hargreaves, 1980) and reinforces their subordinate position in the profession. The positive points mentioned by the students in relation to the teaching staff included:

+Noelle, 3 April 1996, 2nd int., C, 412, 417–424, 432–433
. . . she knows how to put her point across and teach you . . . if she gives you notes, they're well presented, they're well thought out and when she's going through them, it's clear, it's logical, it follows a procedure and she's not afraid to teach us, she doesn't think she's making us lazy by standing up there and teaching … she herself is always studying and she's very good . . .

The negative points made about the tutors were sometimes due to difficulties with interpersonal relationships:

+Jo, 28 March 1996, 2nd int., A, 516–524
. . . it's like being back in secondary school. You know, like, if you don't collect your results the day they're out even though you mightn't even be anywhere near <placename> – 'You have to get your act together' – you know.

This example gives the impression that some teachers do not acknowledge that the students might have other commitments on their time which has been documented as a major source of stress in 53 per cent of midwifery students in the UK (Cavanagh and Snape, 1997).

Some students were taken onto the wards, during classroom time, to do clinical case presentations and this, in common with the findings of other studies (MacLeod, 1995), was universally enjoyed and found to be helpful. There was, however, little clinical teaching by midwives and even simple teaching techniques such as 'teaching the "why" as well as the "how"' (Marson, 1982) were not used.

'Learning to be a midwife'

During the third interviews some students stated that the teaching they had had was too narrow, preparing them for work in their parent hospital alone:

> +Lilian, 13 Nov. 1996, 3rd int., C, 306–320
> <the tutor asked>: 'what types of forceps have you?' and I said 'rotational and non-rotational' 'Oh, my God, where do you get this from?' (gesturing out, shrugging and making a sneering face) . . . you know? There's no such thing as rotational forceps in Hospital C, but there is everywhere else . . . and I'm kind of thinking 'God, according to her I'm wrong, but according to any other place I go, I'm right', so what way do you go?

This is an example of oppressive teaching strategies as outlined by Rather (1994). She maintains that presenting only one side of an issue, as if controversy did not exist, is an attempt to control and intimidate students. Practical midwifery skills were not often taught to the students and many respondents stated, in common with findings of other studies (Chamberlain, 1997), that they learned midwifery skills through trial and error:

> +Nancy, 2 Nov. 1996., 3rd int., D, 299–313
> . . . I remember on number twenty-two delivery only, finding out about assisting the rotation of the baby, and that should have been something you were told straight off. Whatever way the lady had torn and I said: 'God' I said 'what did I do?' because I knew I was going fine until the shoulders came out, the head hadn't torn it at all. And she said to me: 'well, if you'd turned the baby, assisted it round the rotation it wouldn't have happened'. And I said: 'well, thanks a lot!' (sarcastically). Like, this was twenty-two deliveries . . .

The students believed that clinical teaching could take place only in a didactic, teacher led schema involving their removal from the workplace in order to be 'taught'. Bewley maintains that this view 'devalues the teaching role by perpetuating the hierarchy of work, in which service needs come first, and education is abandoned instead of being incorporated.' (Bewley, 1995: 133).

All students had clinical assessments carried out by tutors and a number suggested that these assessments should be included in the final examination. This may be possible in the future as An Bord Altranais has stated that it will recognise the Hospital/University examinations for registration (An Bord Altranais, 1998). The assessment matrix prepared by Fraser et al. (1998) may be useful as a guide for the development of these clinical assessments.

The students found that although they learned how to give routine care, they did not learn the skills of decision making or judgement:

+Isobel, 7 Nov. 1996, 3rd int., C, 269–281
Things might be happening, like . . . a deep transverse arrest, and they'd be talking outside and you'd not be consulted at all. You're there to mind and 'you stay with her now, and if there's a problem you tell us' (frowning, nodding). They don't discuss with you her care or what they're thinking . . .

Cioffi describes how the midwives 'thinking aloud' and vocalising their decision rules may assist students to develop the skills of effective clinical decision making. She also recommends the use of reflection and simulations in developing students' procedural knowledge more rapidly (Cioffi, 1998).

3 Student Midwives' Views of Their Working Role

'It's a whole new ball-game'
In the first few months students found the work and, to some extent, the care that they gave, to be very different from the nursing that they were used to. The change from being a 'staff nurse' to being a 'student' led to a perceived drop in status:

+Jo, 6 July 1995, 1st int., A, 105–108
. . . you are a staff nurse, and yet you're not given the respect of being a staff nurse, you know, you're just back to being a student again.

This reflects the hierarchical nature of nursing, in which status is so hard-won that any slight drop is felt as a backward step, which could decrease job satisfaction (Seymour and Buscherhof, 1991).

'Thrown in the deep end'
The students' overwhelming impression was that they had been plunged into an entirely new world. They were bewildered, lost and unprepared:

+Linda, diary, G, 12–22
My first day was like my first day as a PTS. The nervousness was the same, the butterflies in my stomach; the fact that I was already a qualified

general nurse with two years' experience as a staff nurse in an acute and extremely busy surgical unit was irrelevant. All my previous knowledge seemed to evaporate and counted for very little.

In Ireland, all student midwives must be registered general nurses first although a 'direct entry' programme is an acceptable method of midwife preparation (Council of the EC, 1980). If their general nursing experience is not helpful to them it begs the question: why waste three years undertaking education in the nursing care of ill males and females if one wishes solely to care for childbearing women and their babies?

Almost all the students stated that they had not got sufficient knowledge to cope with the work expected of them in the first few months, findings similar to other areas of midwifery education in the UK (Raymond and Ananda-Rajan, 1993; Chamberlain 1994):

> +Gertie, 11 July 1995, 1st int., C, 382–388
> The worst day would be the first day in delivery on your own with this person and you're told 'go in and do the breathing exercises'. How was I supposed to know what I'm supposed to be doing with breathing exercises?

The responsibility the students were expected to take on seemed, to them, to be enormous, especially as they were left to cope on their own. As one student wrote, in the first verification questionnaire:

> Rebecca, D: It was terrifying looking after a mother in labour not knowing what was normal and abnormal. It was negligence really.

'It's all routine'

In general, the work was described as consisting mainly of tasks, probably because the students were assigned to give the routine, day-to-day care of women which they were capable of doing with little teaching and guidance:

> +Heather, 10 July 95, 1st int., B, 408–415
> . . . you've eighteen women and you're asking them all the same questions 'how are your breasts this morning' and 'are you sore' 'have you gone to the toilet' 'do you want Panadol' and, like, ultimately you know the answers, you know (laughs), they're all going to be the same.

This method of work allocation is a quick and efficient way of training a transient population to give a minimum standard of care (Proctor, 1989). However, qualified staff also conform to the routine (Proctor, 1989) and settle into non-thinking ritualistic ways and students may never learn to plan care in an holistic way, which affects the women in their care (Ball, 1989).

There did not appear to be an emphasis on using research-based practice and some of the practices described had been shown by research to be useless, time–wasting or inadequate:

+Ruth, 13 July 1995, 1st int., D, 754–762
. . . it's just pure task orientated. You do the obs whether they need to be done or not. There's no assessment of whether you could discontinue this, discontinue that. If they've had prolonged rupture of membranes or if they've had a section, they'll have obs here four-hourly until they go home.

'Giving midwifery care'
At the time of the third interviews the majority felt confident in their abilities in certain areas and some complained that they were not given credit for their increased knowledge and experience. Many of the students still professed themselves ignorant of certain procedures:

+Alice, 6 Dec. 1996, 3rd int., E, 147–156
. . . I never thought of assessing how engaged the head was until I saw a senior sister up in the labour ward and . . . she said: 'oh, yeah, she's two-fifths engaged there, you know from your hands'. I'm thinking, here I am – that only happened two months ago – that should have been shown to us a year ago (chopping down with hands).

The staffing levels fell so low that in one hospital the students were taken out of class to work on the wards. Because there was not enough staff to give more relaxed care, the whole point of labour care – to support the woman – became lost in the students' haste to complete expected tasks:

+Noelle, 11 Nov. 1996, 3rd int., C, 309–311
. . . pain relief, you'd love them to take something . . . they make your job more difficult, hanging out of you.

This does not demonstrate the expected 'professional/friend approach' or the 'individualised approach' described by Fraser et al. (1998) as desirable in all qualified midwives. One of the students voiced her own opinion of the way in which maternity care was provided in her hospital:

+Olive, 2 Nov. 1996, 3rd int., D, 841–849
It's like this rotary belt you know, get her labour going, get the baby out, get her downstairs, get the other woman in, get this thing going (gesturing on each phrase). It's losing the personal touch and it's not allowing the woman to be herself and to labour in her own way.

This 'depersonalization' of birth (Kitzinger, 1992) has reduced what used to be a significant phase in human life to a mere physiological process under the command and direction of medical 'experts'.

4 Student Midwives' Views of Relationships with Staff

'Them and us'

Many respondents commented on the perceived gap between the status of staff and of students which has also been described in other studies (Kiger, 1993). This was particularly obvious in the labour wards:

+Olive, 13 July 1995, 1st int., D, 438–441, 446–450
. . . there's . . . a very definite line between staff and student . . . we have our own little tea room as such and they have their tea room. Totally separate, like, you don't relate to them, there's a very definite line there.

The work that they were assigned to do often involved 'non-nursing' tasks, or nursing tasks that they knew how to do already; consequently they felt that they were not learning any new clinical skills. The Council of the European Communities' Directive on midwifery education states unequivocally that students 'shall be taught the responsibilities involved in the activities of midwives' (Council of the EC, 1980: 3) which is difficult to do if they are performing different duties.

'They all have their moments'

The majority of students spoke of an unwelcoming atmosphere and seemed to find their initial relations with qualified staff unhelpful:

+Corrie, diary, F, 48–54
Example, at 3.45 p.m. (end of shift), I went up to desk (sister and senior staff sitting there) and asked if I could go off duty to get a 'dirty' look and a grunt for an answer – so I presume that means yes and went, because after all I was off duty.

Students who work in an unfriendly atmosphere do not learn as much as when they are relaxed enough to build a rapport with staff (Marson, 1982) or when they feel 'safe to ask questions' (Fretwell, 1983). Some senior staff were sarcastic, put the students down and belittled them, often in front of others, all behaviours which have been shown to cause stress and hinder student nurse learning (Wong, 1978; Birch, 1983; Campbell et al., 1994).

Students received support and encouragement from other students. They used passive methods of coping and avoided confrontation with those in authority, submissive conduct which demonstrates oppressed group behaviour (Roberts, 1983):

+Alice, 2 Aug. 1995, 1st int., E, 164–170
'. . . don't bath baby like that', I don't bath baby like that – end of story; I'm told 'don't start the beds 'til after second break', I don't start the beds 'til after second break; 'stay in your own section', I stay in my own section . . .

These reactions are similar to those expressed by students in other studies who accepted difficulties passively (Wynne et al., 1993) and concentrated on 'getting through' (Melia, 1981; Pilhammar Andersson, 1995). This pressure to conform was also found in Pollert's study of young female factory workers who worked under the constant threat of demotion unless they kept up their production level (Pollert, 1981). There appear to be many similarities between the conditions of factory workers and student midwives which emphasise the existence of an industrial model of childbirth provision.

'Knowing your place'

The majority of students believed that they had a lowly place in the acknowledged hierarchy of the midwifery profession:

> +Eleanor, 1 April 1996, 2nd int., A, 607–610
> . . . little things, no tea break for the students, the staff get one . . . you
> have to watch your time, you get a half hour or whatever, they take an
> hour and a half . . .

This two-tier system of allocation of work and breaks is very divisive and may also be seen as a form of bullying in that it is an 'abuse of power . . . which makes the recipient feel . . . upset . . .' (RCM, 1996: 3). The routine, rules and regulations of the hospital also served to keep students 'in their place':

> +Lee, 13 March 1996, 2nd int., A, 338–346
> . . . I was on night duty and we're supposed to get off at a quarter past
> eight and we kind of said, well, one of us can go at ten past eight and . . .
> the sister in charge on nights told me I was coming off night duty two
> minutes too early, she sent me back.

Du Toit noted that students' values, behaviour and concepts of self change as professional socialisation occurs , so that all students eventually become like the staff (Du Toit, 1995). One student in this study also identified this continuous, reinforcing circle:

> +Cecilia, 1 May 1996, 2nd int., C, 556–562
> Cecilia: Oh yes, the tutors laugh and say we'll do the same, you know:
>   'we've heard those complaints for years and years and you'll turn
>   around and do the same yourself.'
> C.B.: That's sad, isn't it?
> Cecilia: It's like dry rot.

Using reflective diaries as an educational tool may assist those students, once qualified, to remember how it felt to be a learner (Schon, 1983).

'There's a definite hierarchy'

It had become clear from discussions with all students during the third interviews that a hierarchical system (Hugman, 1991) was in operation in the majority of maternity hospitals:

+Ciara, 6 Dec. 1996, 3rd int., E, 241–251
And these are people working for, like, 25 years. Imagine the carry-on, imagine at that stage of your life you're still bowing and minding out of the way, 'sister's coming!' (whispering). It's hilarious, grown women that are organising families and everything, a whole weight of problems on their shoulders, coming in and suddenly being walked all over by someone by the colour of the uniform they wear.

Carlisle maintains that midwives are under extreme stress due to a mismatch between being educated to be autonomous practitioners and then practising in an institutional setting where they are not free to make their own decisions (Carlisle et al., 1994). This causes frustration which may then be taken out on students:

Group interview, Hospital G
Student: I actually woke up one morning and discovered bruises on my arm where a staff nurse had grabbed me and pulled me out of delivery room. And she said to me: 'the least you could have done was to have the caps off the Zylocaine, ready for Doctor X'. I nearly died . . .

Some hospitals had rigid policies concerning sick leave, which required students to present a medical certificate for even one day's illness. Those students who had had to take sick leave or time off for bereavements were not always sympathetically received:

Anonymous, third interview
. . . on the morning of the funeral I got a phone-call from my Matron to get back to work, that my patient came first, and that my cousin who had died was only a first cousin and it didn't matter, despite the fact that it was a sudden death at 21 (face grim, twisting hands).

These accounts illustrate the lack of caring shown to those in the caring professions by their 'superiors' in the hierarchy. The problem with this type of attitude is that being uncared for makes people uncaring for others (Grigsby and Megel, 1995).

CONCLUSIONS AND RECOMMENDATIONS

The 13 weeks allocated for theoretical input on the midwifery education programme in Southern Ireland is far too short. Students need time to acquire adult learning skills, to have an increased amount of clinical teaching and to develop their critical thinking and judgement. Theoretical teaching needs to be broadened and thought given to the integration of theory and practice.

In the clinical areas, opportunities for staff to teach and explain decisions while giving care should be identified and utilised. The use of prepared mentors, sufficient support staff to undertake non-midwifery duties and a more caring approach to all staff will aid students in their education.

It appears that midwifery care in Ireland, as described by these students, is governed not by a midwifery model, or even by a medical one, but by an economic or industrial model which lays stress on swift throughput of clients. Staffing levels should be examined and the use of routines and non-research based care should be phased out. Students need to be assisted, with support from educated mentors, to plan care in an holistic way which will enable them to develop their midwifery skills in the future. This will result in improved, empowering care for the women of Ireland.

ACKNOWLEDGEMENTS

I thank the students involved for their wholehearted enthusiasm and interest. Thanks are also due to the Matrons and Principal Tutors in the seven hospitals who granted permission for the study to be conducted. Financial support for part of this study was gratefully received from the Royal College of Surgeons in Ireland, An Bord Altranais and Gillespie Ltd.

NOTE

1   The Ethnograph V4.0, Qualis Research Associates, P.O. Box 2070, Amherst, MA 01004, 413–256–8835

REFERENCES

Alexander, M. F. (1983) *Learning to Nurse*. Edinburgh: Churchill Livingstone.

Ashworth, P. D. and Longmate, M. A. (1993) Theory and practice: beyond the dichotomy, *Nurse Education Today*, 13: 321–7.

Ball, J. (1989) Postnatal care and adjustment to motherhood, in: S. Robinson and A. Thomson (eds), *Midwives, Research and Childbirth*, Vol. 1. London: Chapman & Hall: 154–75.

Begley, C. M. (1996) Using triangulation in nursing research, *Journal of Advanced Nursing*, 24 (1): 122–8.

Begley, C. M. (1997) Midwives in the making: A longitudinal study of the experiences of student midwives during their two-year training in Ireland, unpublished PhD thesis, Trinity College, University of Dublin.

Begley, C. M. (1998) Student midwives' experiences in the first three months of their training: 'good days and bad days', *Nursing Review*, 16 (3/4): 77–81.

Begley, C. M. (1999a) A study of student midwives' experiences during their two-year education programme, *Midwifery* (in press).

Begley, C. M. (1999b) Student midwives' views of the working role during midwifery training: 'Thrown in at the deep end', *Nursing Review*, 17(3): 76–81.

Begley, C. M. (1999c) Student midwives views of 'learning to be a midwife' in Ireland, *Midwifery* (in press).

Bewley, C. (1995) Clinical teaching in midwifery – an exploration of meanings, *Nurse Education Today*, 15: 129–35.

Birch, J. (1983) Anxiety and conflict in nurse education, in: B. Davis (ed), *Research into Nurse Education*. London: Croom Helm: 26–47

An Bord Altranais (1998) *Nurses Rules 1988 (Amendment) Rules 1998 – Explanatory Memorandum*. Circular no. 6 Dublin: An Bord Altranais.

Byrne, U. (1989) Family planning information: the contribution of the midwife. Unpublished BNS thesis. University College Dublin.

Campbell, I. E., Larrivee, L., Field, P. A., Day, R. A., and Reutter, L. (1994) Learning to nurse in the clinical setting, *Journal of Advanced Nursing*, 20: 1125–31.

Carlisle, C., Baker, G. A., Riley, M., and Dewey, M. (1994) Stress in midwifery: a comparison of midwives and nurses using the work environment scale, *International Journal of Nursing Studies*, 31: 13–22.

Cavanagh, S. J. and Snape, J. (1997) Educational sources of stress in midwifery students, *Nurse Education Today*, 17: 128–34.

Chamberlain, M. (1994) Factors affecting the acquisition of skills in midwifery students. Unpublished PhD thesis. University of London.

Chamberlain, M. (1997) Challenges of clinical learning for student midwives, *Midwifery*, 13: 85–91.

Cioffi, J. (1998) Education for clinical decision making in midwifery practice, *Midwifery*, 14: 18–22.

Coleman, H. (1989) Transition to motherhood: a study of the experience of primiparous mothers in the six weeks following discharge from maternity hospital. Unpublished BNS thesis. University College Dublin.

Coughlan, M. (1995) The hidden curriculum in nurse education. Unpublished MEd thesis. University College Dublin.

Council of the European Communities (1980) *Council Directive 80/155/EEC, No. L33/8*. Brussels: Council of the European Communities.

Davies, R. M. (1990) Perspectives on midwifery: students' beginnings, *Research and the Midwife Conference Proceedings 1990*. Manchester, 1990: 37–48.

Department of Health (1976) Statistical information relevant to the health services. Dublin: Stationery Office.

Donnison, J. (1988) *Midwives and Medical Men: A History of the Struggle for the Control of Childbirth*. London: Historical Publications.

Du Toit, D. (1995) A sociological analysis of the extent and influence of professional socialization on the development of a nursing identity among nursing students at two universities in Brisbane, Australia, *Journal of Advanced Nursing*, 21: 164–71.

Field, P.A. and Morse, J. (1985) *Nursing Research: The Application of Qualitative Approaches*. London: Croom Helm.

Fretwell, J. (1983) Creating a ward learning environment: the sister's role, *Nursing Times*, Occasional Papers 79: 21–2.

Fraser, D., Murphy, R. and Worth-Butler, M. (1998) *Preparing Effective Midwives: An Outcome Evaluation of the Effectiveness of Pre-Registration Midwifery Programmes of Education*. London: English National Board for Nursing, Midwifery and Health Visiting.

Golden, J. (1980) Midwifery training: The views of newly qualified midwives, *Midwives Chronicle and Nursing Notes*, 93 (1109): 190–4.

Greenwood, J. (1993) The apparent desensitization of student nurses during their professional socialization: a cognitive perspective, *Journal of Advanced Nursing*, 18: 1471—79.

Grigsby, K. A. and Megel, M. E. (1995) Caring experiences of nurse educators, *Journal of Nursing Education*, 34: 411–18.

Hargreaves, D. (1980) Power and the paracurriculum, in: A. Finch and P. Scrimshaw (eds), *Standards, Schooling and Education*. Sevenoaks, Kent: Hodder & Stoughton.

Holloway, I. and Wheeler, S. (1996) *Qualitative Research for Nurses*. Oxford: Blackwell: 126–37.

Hugman, R. (1991) *Power in Caring Professions*. London: Macmillan.

Kiger, A. M. (1993) Accord and discord in students' images of nursing, *Journal of Nursing Education*, 32 (7): 309–17.

Kitzinger, S. (1992) *Ourselves as Mothers*. London: Doubleday.

Macleod, M. L. P. (1995) What does it mean to be well taught? A hermeneutic course evaluation, *Journal of Nursing Education*, 34: 197–203.

Marson, S. N. (1982) Ward sister – teacher or facilitator? An investigation into the behavioural characteristics of effective ward teachers, *Journal of Advanced Nursing*, 7: 347–57.

May, N., Veitch, L., Mcintosh, J. B., and Alexander, M. F. (1997) *Evaluation of Nurse and Midwife Education in Scotland*. Glasgow: Glasgow Caledonian University.

McCaugherty, D. (1991) The theory-practice gap in nurse education: its causes and possible solutions. Findings from an action research study, *Journal of Advanced Nursing*, 16: 1055–61.

Melia, K. M. (1981) Student nurses' accounts of their work and training: a qualitative analysis. Unpublished PhD thesis. University of Edinburgh

Murphy-Lawless, J. (1991) Piggy in the middle: the midwife's role in achieving woman-controlled childbirth, *The Irish Journal of Psychology*, 12: 198–215.

Murphy-Lawless, J. (1998) *Reading Birth and Death: A History of Obstetric Thinking*. Cork: Cork University Press.

Pilhammar Andersson, E. (1995) Marginality: concept or reality in nursing education? *Journal of Advanced Nursing*, 21: 131–6.

Pollert, A. (1981) *Girls, Wives and Factory Lives*. London: Macmillan.

Proctor, S. (1989) The functioning of nursing routines in the management of a transient workforce, *Journal of Advanced Nursing*, 14: 184–5.

Rather, M. L. (1994) Schooling for oppression: a critical hermeneutical analysis of the lived experience of the returning RN student, *Journal of Nursing Education*, 33 (6): 268–9.

Raymond, J. and Ananda-Rajan, K. (1993) Learning practice, *Nursing Times*, 89: 36–7.

Roberts, S. J. (1983) Oppressed behaviour: implications for nursing, *Advances in Nursing Science*, 5: 21–30.

Robinson, S. (1986) Midwifery training: the views of newly qualified midwives, *Nurse Education Today*, 6: 49–59.

Robinson, S. (1991) Preparation for practice: The educational experience and career intentions of newly qualified midwives, in: S. Robinson and A. M. Thomson (eds), *Midwives, Research and Childbirth*, Vol. 2. London: Chapman & Hall: 8–41.

Royal College of Midwives (1996) *In Place of Fear.* London: Royal College Of Midwives.

Schon, D. (1983) *The Reflective Practitioner: How Professionals Think in Action.* New York: Basic Books.

Seed, A. (1991) Becoming a registered nurse: the student's perspective. Unpublished PhD thesis. Leeds Polytechnic.

Seymour, E. and Buscherhof, J. R. (1991) Sources and consequences of satisfaction and dissatisfaction in nursing: findings from a national sample, *International Journal of Nursing Studies*, 28 (2): 109–24.

Smith, P. (1987) The relationship between quality of nursing care and the ward as a learning environment: developing a methodology, *Journal of Advanced Nursing*, 12 (4): 413–20.

Treacy, M. P. (1987) 'In the pipeline': a qualitative study of general nurse training with special reference to nurses' role in health education. Unpublished PhD thesis. University of London.

Wagner, M. (1994) *Pursuing the birth machine: The search for appropriate birth technology.* Camperdown: ACE Graphics.

Wiley, M. M. and Merriman, B. (1996) *Women and health care in Ireland.* Dublin: Oak Tree Press.

Wilson, A., Startup, R. (1991) Nurse socialization: issues and problems, *Journal of Advanced Nursing*, 16: 1478–86.

Wong, S. (1978) Nurse-teacher behaviours in the clinical field: apparent effect on nursing students' learning, *Journal of Advanced Nursing*, 3: 369–72.

Wynne, R., Clarkin, N., and McNieve A. (1993) *The Experience of Stress amongst Irish Nurses – A Survey of Irish Nurses' Organisation Members.* Dublin: Irish Nurses' Organisation.

Notes on Contributors

Cecily M. Begley is a registered general nurse, midwife and midwife teacher. She is currently the Director of the School of Nursing and Midwifery Studies at Trinity College, Dublin. Her research interests include physiological childbirth, nursing and midwifery education and self-esteem and assertiveness in nurses and midwives.

Janice Clarke is a registered general nurse currently practising as a lecturer in the School of Nursing and Midwifery, University of Southampton. She has extensive experience in curriculum development and its operation at pre and post registration levels with particular skills in accreditation of prior and experiential learning. Her teaching responsibilities encompass undergraduate research education and clinical supervision together with qualitative research approaches for multidisciplinary postgraduate students. Her research interests focus on multidisciplinary values of caring, currently in the field of neuro-disability, to inform educational preparation for caring practices.

Rita Collins is a lecturer in the School of Nursing and Midwifery at University College Dublin. Her principal teaching and research interests centre on the areas of education of nurses, patient education, assessment methodologies and nursing informatics.

Mary Farrelly is a psychiatric nurse working in An Bord Altranais as a project assistant to Scope of Nursing and Midwifery Practice Project on secondment from her post as a nursing practice development coordinator. Her research interests include quality in health care particularly from patients' perspectives and the role of the psychiatric nurse in the health service.

Gerard M. Fealy is a lecturer in School of Nursing and Midwifery, University College Dublin. He has a background in medical and coronary care nursing. He has worked as a nurse tutor at St James's Hospital,

Dublin, and was formerly principal nurse tutor at Our Lady of Lourdes Hospital, Drogheda. He has published numerous papers in the Irish and international academic press and his current research interests include research priorities and research utilisation, curriculum policy and practice and the history of nurse education in Ireland.

Mary Gobbi is a lecturer in nursing at the University of Southampton, specialising in education, policy and management. Her particular interests are the learning and development of nurses in practice, the relationships between the epistemological and ontological in practice and the associated methodological challenges posed when researching both 'at home' and 'away'. She is currently working on projects dealing with staff retention and nurses returning to practice.

Abbey Hyde has a background in nursing and sociology. She is currently a lecturer in the School of Nursing and Midwifery at University College Dublin, having previously lectured at the University of Edinburgh. Her doctoral research completed in 1996 was on the pregnancy experiences of single mothers. Her research interests include the politics of reproduction, nursing practices in relation to older people and the initiation of smoking in adolescence.

Geraldine McCarthy is Professor of Nursing and Director of the Department of Nursing Studies at University College Cork since its establishment in 1994. She has established a number of programmes and is active in reasearch. She has held a number of nursing positions in Ireland the UK, USA and Canada.

Hugh McKenna is Professor of Nursing and Head of the School of Health Sciences at the University of Ulster and also Nurse Commissioner at the Southern Health and Social Services Board. He has published over 65 journal articles and written and co-written four books. He is Assistant Editor of *Quality of Health Care* and the *International Journal of Nursing Studies* and an editorial board member of four other journals. He is involved in research into a range of nursing phenomena including primary care and nursing skill mix.

Therese Connell Meehan is a lecturer in the School of Nursing and Midwifery at University College Dublin. She received her initial nursing education in New Zealand, and has a BScN from the University of Pennsylvania and an MA and PhD in Nursing from New York University. She has practised in medical-surgical and maternal-child nursing and was Director of the Nursing Research Programme at New York University

Medical Center for several years. Her special interests include palliative nursing, integrating research and practice, conceptual model and theory development, the spiritual dimension of nursing and nursing history.

Laserina O'Connor is a lecturer in the School of Nursing and Midwifery, University College Dublin. Her speciality is critical care and diabetes nursing She has a special interest in pain assessment, documentation and management within the context of critical care nursing.

Aine O'Meara Kearney is a registered general nurse and has held positions in clinical nursing, nurse education and nursing management. She is currently working as a member of a multidisciplinary team, facilitating quality improvement in patient administration services in the acute hospital sector. Her research interests include change management, nursing practice development and skillmix/workload measurement.

Kader Parahoo is Senior Lecturer in the School of Health Sciences at the University of Ulster. His background is in nursing, health promotion and sociology. He has published a number of articles on research issues and methodology and is the author of *Nursing Research: Principles, Process and Issues* (Macmillan, 1997). His main interests are in evidence-based practice and research utilisation.

Sam Porter has eight years' experience of clinical practice as a general nurse, and eight years' experience of lecturing in sociology at Queen's University, Belfast. He is currently the Professor of Nursing Research in the School of Nursing and Midwifery at Queen's. His publications range across the disciplines of sociology and nursing.

Kathy Redmond is a lecturer in the School of Nursing and Midwifery, University College Dublin. She is joint editor of *Cancer in the Elderly: A Nursing and Medical Perspective* (Elsevier, 1997) and joint author of *Pain: Causes and Management* (Blackwell Science, 1998). Her interests include symptom management, clinical decision making and patient participation in care and she has published widely on these topics. She was President of the European Oncology Nursing Society, 1993–97, and is currently education coordinator and executive board member of this Society.

Helen Simons, Professor of Education at the University of Southampton, is a specialist in evaluation who has published widely in the field of qualitative methodology, case study and the ethics of research. She has directed numerous research projects including the external independent evaluation of the Registration/Diploma Nurse Education and Training

programme in Ireland and the training of evaluators to evaluate
educational reform in Poland. Currently she is a member of the Research
and Development Group of the English national Board for Nursing,
Midwifery and Health Visiting and the Executive Council of the UK
Evaluation Society.

Margaret P. Treacy is Head of the School of Nursing and Midwifery at
University College Dublin. She was awarded a PhD from the University
of London in 1987 for her study of the learning experiences of a group
of general nursing students in Ireland. She has engaged in extensive
curriculum development work and is currently undertaking research on
young people and smoking, and nurses' role in health promotion. She is
on the editorial boards of the *International Journal of Nursing Practice* and
the *Medico-Legal Journal of Ireland*.

Roger Watson entered nursing from a background in the biological
sciences. After specialising in the care of older people, he moved to the
Department of Nursing Studies at the University of Edinburgh. He has
published widely in the biological sciences applied to nursing, geron-
tology and caring in nursing. After leaving Edinburgh he worked in
Ireland and is now Professor of Nursing at the University of Hull, England.

Index